Getting at
the Root

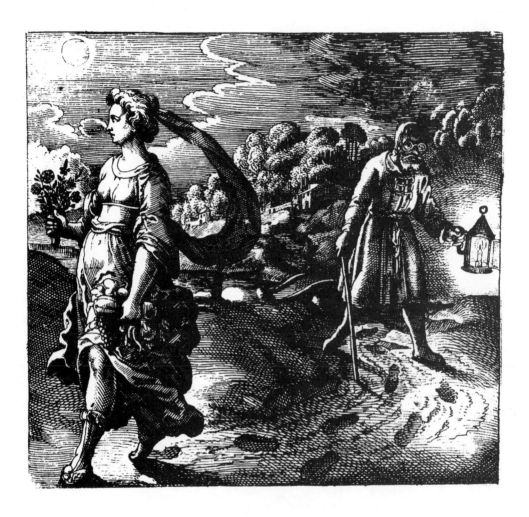

Nature be your guide; follow her with your art willingly, closely.
You err, if she is not your companion on your way.
Reason be your staff. Exercise may strengthen your sight,
On account of which things that are far away can be discerned.
Literature be your lamp, shining in the darkness,
In order to guard you against an accumulation of things and words.

—Michael Maier

Getting at the Root

Treating the Deepest Source of Disease

ANDREW LANGE, N.D.

North Atlantic Books
Berkeley, California

Published by
North Atlantic Books
P.O. Box 12327
Berkeley, California 94712

Cover and book design by Jennifer Dunn

Printed in the United States of America

Getting at the Root: Treating the Deepest Source of Disease is sponsored by the Society for the Study of Native Arts and Sciences, a nonprofit educational corporation whose goals are to develop an educational and crosscultural perspective linking various scientific, social, and artistic fields; to nurture a holistic view of arts, sciences, humanities, and healing; and to publish and distribute literature on the relationship of mind, body, and nature.

North Atlantic Books are available through most bookstores. To contact North Atlantic directly, call 800-337-2665 or visit our website at www.northatlanticbooks.com.

Substantial discounts on bulk quantities of North Atlantic books are available to corporations, professional associations, and other organizations. For details and discount information, contact the special sales department at North Atlantic Books.

LIBRARY OF CONGRESS CATALOGING-IN-PUBLICATION DATA

Lange, Andrew, 1957–
    Getting at the root : treating the deepest source of disease / by Andrew Lange.
        p. ; cm.
Includes bibliographical references.
    ISBN 1-55643-395-6 (pbk.)
1. Homeopathy. 2. Vitalism.
    [DNLM: 1. Homeopathy. 2. Holistic Health. 3. Medicine, Traditional. 4. Vitalism. WB 930 L274g 2002] I. Title.

RX71 .L36 2002
615.5'32—dc21

                                                                    2002005811

                1   2   3   4   5   6   7   /   06   05   04   03   02

Contents

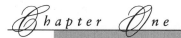

Chapter One

A Geography of Medicine

If you can look into the seeds of time,
And say which seed will grow and which will not,
Then speak to me.

—William Shakespeare

Finding the Principles

This book is an investigation of the myths of science and natural medicine. It engages a vitalistic philosophy, in which our study of the body views consciousness as the central influence on physiology. It incorporates metaphor and history to confirm our work. It is the acknowledgment of mutually unique perceptions of the world that can contribute to resolving inner conflict and disease. We bring our experience and tradition to understand the healing power of nature. It is supported by observation in clinical practice and in life. This is one history, one story, which reminds us of what we were never told, that we already know.

We live as if we know. We think we understand what others mean. We believe our dreams will come to fruition. Yet our lives reach beyond the limitations of our perceptions. Our bodies are a pool of neural responses and sensory reflections that contains the potential of our imaginations and maintains the ground of our pain and joy. If what we knew about life or maintained as our philosophy could explain its sheer mystery, perhaps we would be more capable of addressing our suffering. But we are guided by a mere thread of experiences, linked together by common elements and maintained by parameters of familiarity that we have created and agreed upon.

It is our disease that demands we turn our attention to the course we have taken. The suffering of our disease demands that we question how we live our lives. The question may be about what enters our bodies, or how we communicate and interact. We may discover a structural defect, or a trait transferred through our family. The source may be a poison or simply a mistranslation through which we have built a defense that is no longer appropriate or necessary. Disease speaks of something we have forgotten, ignored, or simply been unaware of.

Disease and medicine do not exist as polarities. Disease is an information system, a feedback mechanism. It tells us what we have ignored. The symptoms are an inherent mechanism to make us aware of the problem. Like a warning light, symptoms indicate the inner problem. In and of themselves they are not the cause. The origins may be in the body or they may exist as a disease of the community. Like a virus, the hidden source of our illness may remain latent in a single cell or be expressed through the entire system. Most importantly, the changes generated through illness may operate to the detriment of health, or they may contribute to evolution and adaptation.

If we see disease and medicine as opposites, we fail to respect the intelligence of natural homeostatic systems that act to protect us psychologically and physically. These lacks of insight lead to implement methods that may suppress the organisms' own attempts to heal. We try to overcome disease, overcome the body and overcome nature. It is our fears that lead us to react to the response rather than seeking its source.

The tendency to simplify disease and its treatment may occur whether the approach utilizes herbs, chemicals, or words. Whether treatment leads to a lasting cure is determined by the manner in which we address the disease. It is a question of how we aid or interfere in the healing process. The body is more intelligent than the doctor. Though medicine has progressed tremendously, we still have very old beliefs as well as newly emerging cultural expectations that maintain their power over how we see our own treatment. We rationalize our failures or displace the responsibility of cure to rely on the efficacy of the placebo response.

The archetype of the healer is a cultural image. We may believe in the doctor with the white coat or the medicine man who lives far from society. So much of the efficacy of treatment depends on its acceptance by the patient. This is not absolutely necessary for the treatment to work; however, it is critical to maintain compliance and sustain continuity in the relationship of care.

Our method of treatment reflects the depth of our understanding of the nature of disease, and the corresponding effect should be a catalyst for a sustained level of change. It must be evaluated in the context of how we understand the unfoldment of the healing process. The goal of treatment could be a singular act in the context of a lifelong process of transformation. It is an unwinding and release of old unresolved ailments, and the process of enhancing our capacity for regeneration. This is only possible through our attention to the ignored details.

The initial cry becomes a whisper. The longer the message is sent without being heard, the weaker its transmission and more vague its interpretation. Many of our drugs simply act to suppress the symptom until it is masked or forgotten, as if we could hide something under the bed and no one would ever know, not even ourselves.

We are left with wastebasket diagnoses, which tell us little of either their origins or treatment. A wastebasket diagnosis is a superficial one in which the individual's condition is generalized into a syndrome, such as chronic fatigue or hyperactivity, a category that may fit insurance billing without really describing the suffering of the patient. Through extensive testing our disease may be categorized in an attempt to group common symptoms when the mechanism is unknown, with no cure in sight. Often we find blood tests that border statistical norms, but don't fit into a clear diagnosis.

This is where the term idiopathic is applied, meaning the cause is unknown. Fatigue and malaise, shifting pains that metastasize in patterns that defy definition, autoimmune disorders, and hysteria are all hallmarks of a confused system that lacks the vitality and organization to express its disease with clarity.

Vitalistic Medicine

One of the most difficult aspects of understanding any system of healing is to gain an understanding of its goals. The traditional systems of medicine have maintained the most integrated examples of vitalistic and decentralized methods.

By traditional, I mean systems that have a coherent philosophical and cultural history. Traditional methods have endured the changing opinions of medical experimentation. The dominant practice of medicine represents an orthodoxy, but not necessarily a tradition.

[4]

In a vitalistic approach, we recognize the larger influences that inhabit cultural, environmental, and spiritual domains. Vitalism recognizes a capacity for the organism to self-regulate, to maintain or reestablish homeostasis under the appropriate conditions. Vitalism represents the philosophy of a life force. It sees a world in which the whole is larger than the sum of its parts, with a central regulation of the organism by consciousness. Vitalistic medicine is therefore a method that draws upon the body's own ability to heal itself.

In a decentralized system, we value a science that searches for health care that is appropriate for the community it serves, respecting the needs of the individual, and engaging them in their own attempts to heal.

In engaging the concepts of vitalism, I am not suggesting that the phenomenon of life is inexplicable in terms of natural science, but that the complexity of biological systems requires more than reductionist approaches. Historically, vitalism has been an attempt to engage the life force or soul in the treatment of disease. Since science has overwhelmingly rejected the possibility of such influences by isolating the description of human life solely to its physiological models, vitalistic methods have been ignored or condemned. The recognition of the spiritual as an influence on mankind has been untenable in a scientific model. Though we now are capable of describing at least ten dimensions of existence mathematically, our biological sciences remain engaged in the proofs of three dimensions.

Vitalistic thought is not opposed to these descriptions. To find a deeper understanding of life, modern vitalism has to be engaged with its counterparts in science. Rather than stating itself as a science, vitalism is an investigation of all sciences, including the forgotten, the misinterpreted and the hidden. The scientific method that has come to dominate modern medicine is only one representation of science. It ignores what is beyond its method. It ignores any language that is outside itself. It represents a powerful but isolated world that refuses to speak or even recognize any other language.

The roots and branches of these arguments have deep traditions. The early historical philosophies of medicine can still be seen in today's practice. The Roman physician Galen was a surgeon whose influence persists in modern medicine. His method pervaded the Dark Ages almost exclusively, continuing until the Renaissance. He defined a system in which disease is to be counteracted. Disease is still widely seen as something that is to be removed, not understood.

[5]

Tradition and Orthodoxy

The course of modern medicine has become an orthodoxy. It does not exist solely as allopathy, the use of medicines to attack disease. Orthodox medicine has become much too sophisticated to be described as a singular approach. However, it has become energy-intensive, in that it imposes the most complex approaches, when simpler solutions may suffice. This is not because of a lack of knowledge of physiology, rather it is a dependence on treatments to overcome physiology instead of enhancing the body's own physiological function. It is a medicine influenced by economics, patenting, and business that uses science as a language. Though allopathic medicine has its own strong tradition, its application in modern society is often driven by an expediency that can ignore consistent medical principles in the need for immediate effect.

In many cases, traditional medicines have provided answers that orthodox methods have failed to solve. An example of this is the treatment of hepatitis, which has been successfully treated in every major traditional medical system, with the exception of Western orthodoxy.

Traditional medicine functions to enhance a sense of belonging, to the body, to the environment, and to the community. Traditional methods are certainly not universal in their ability to treat disease. Both Tradition and Orthodoxy risk the creating of a hierarchy, in which the patient is a mystified believer in the superior knowledge of the medical pundits.

Every method of healing has an intention of curing. However, the definition of cure can be very different, depending upon the depth of perspective in which the context of disease and cure are seen.

People speak today of "energy medicine." We cannot divide physiology and energy in understanding our bodies. Much of the language of energetics can be simply another description of attempts to manipulate physiology. Certainly when we talk about physiology, or the body, we are talking about energy. Whether it is the churning of metabolism and enzymatic expressions of the cell, or a smile, it is the movement and expression of energy.

When we understand the forces acting behind the reaction, then we understand its energetic dimension.

It is surprising that the public often places all of natural therapeutics under the name of Eastern medicine. Similarly, the common expression of Western medicine is assumed to solely represent Orthodox medicine. This misperception may be due to the lack of a sufficient number of accredited schools teaching Western traditions of natural medicine, or it may simply reflect an inherent fascination with exotic foreign systems. These systems are rich and fascinating, but the approach taken here is to understand the Western tradition of medicine. The understanding of energetics must apply to both systems. In Western medicine the concepts of energetics have largely been studied in relation to spiritual forms of healing. Though the study of medicines and therapeutics from an energetic perspective may be threatening to the dominant paradigm, the contributions they offer for the integration of mind and body in medicine are crucial.

Through understanding the Western traditions, we can find potentials that remain latent in our own indigenous medicines and culture. Ultimately, we can understand how medicine and healing interact in a language that supersedes categorization and individual systems. Although homeopathy is utilized in this book as a primary model of vitalistic medicine, my goal is to explore questions surrounding health care beyond any singular approach so that a more broad understanding of the underlying philosophies can help us to evaluate the treatment we receive.

Early systems of medicine are often romantically divined solely as energy medicine as much as they are cast aside as primitive. In fact, neither is accurate. Early civilizations made great contributions to the practice of medicine, some of which was incorporated, some of which was lost. The humoral systems of medicine, such as early Greek medicine, Chinese medicine, and Ayurveda use both methods to enhance healing and opposing treatments to control symptoms. The divisions of mechanism and vitalism still exist in these systems, even though they speak in energetic terms.

In humoral systems diseases are divided into hot, cold, dry, or wet. A hot disease requires a cold treatment. A wet disease needs drying influences. The intended view is to bring the body into balance. This may lead to a dependency on treatments to maintain balance, rather than the medicine's ability to reeducate the system as a whole.

The strength of the humoral system is that it brings forth a greater reliance on the ability of treatment to facilitate function, to engage the body's own systems. These include improving the capacities for the kidneys, liver, and skin to eliminate waste products and toxins. It induces the ability for the body to produce fevers and respond immunologically. Even today the term humoral is used in immunology to describe the aspect of our immune system that acts systemically throughout the body in the serum of the blood and lymph glands, rather than the cellular level.

Eastern methods have influenced Western ideas throughout history. Vedic Medicine of India and Arabic Medicine were primary influences on the development of Greek Medicine and thought. Chinese medicine is not new to the West. Athanasius Kircher introduced Chinese medicine in 1667, in his book, *China Illustrata*. Articles on Ginseng, the great Asian panacea or adaptogen, appeared in medical journals from the 1830s. In the nineteenth century, wild American ginseng was largely traded to China.

Today many of the early insights that understood the spiritual basis of disease in early Chinese medicine have degenerated into mechanical treatments, with the energetic language left intact. In the case of China, much of the historical tradition was considered antagonistic to the goals of the government, due to its spiritual foundations, and were repressed by Chairman Mao during the Cultural Revolution.

In China, the materialistic thought under Communist rule and the demands of treating large populations have transformed much of the focus of herbal treatments toward immediate results. In treating epidemic diseases, such as flus and infections, this was largely appropriate and effective. But understanding the source of disease it is not always as clear.

The Chinese medical philosophy has a saying: "Treat the root and the stem (or periphery)." In practice both are often attempted at the same time to assure recovery. This runs the risk of acting in contradictory ways. If we view symptoms as the body's attempt to maintain homeostasis, then the treatment of superficial symptoms may actually suppress the body's capacity to mount an adequate response to other compromised systems in the body, or to future disease influences.

Theoretically, the goal is to find the central influence of the disease condition. Diagnosis becomes the key. In the vitalistic tradition, treatment and its effectiveness will depend on what its source is determined to be.

What is the root of disease? In chronic disease it becomes more complicated. It is negligent to treat superfical diagnosis, or common syndromes in Chinese medicine, such as liver fire or weak kidney yin, without understanding the emerging hidden cancer or diabetes.

The chronic persistence of infections and their effects is a commonly misdiagnosed aspect of disease. The broad descriptions of an infection in humoral systems as "internal heat or fire" may be too generalized and obfuscate a more accurate diagnosis and treatment.

The weakness in all systems of medicine is inaccurate or superficial diagnoses, which lead to an inappropriate treatment or dependency on continued inadequate care. Often the patient is led through a series of treatments without a clear sense of outcome. In autopsy studies, Orthodox medicine has been proven to be more inaccurate in diagnosis of post-mortem autopsies; though it should be their greatest strength.

In any medical system, the philosophical principles can be compromised in clinical application. The demands and beliefs of the patient or the culture can define what the practitioner can offer.

[9]

MECHANICS AND ENERGETICS

It is important to see that any system can be applied energetically or mechanically, whether it is plant-based medicine or surgery. The removal of a tumor may free tremendous amounts of fixated energy in the body. If the central theme of holism is the interaction of mind and body, then the weapon we wield must not create further defenses, and must be capable of addressing the influence that generated the disease in the first place.

We can assess the comparative depth of treatment by finding which method addresses the patient's awareness. This is where we may find the meaning of disease, the patient's mythology as to why they suffer. Rather than just applying our diagnostic system, we need to hear what is being said. The person might not even be capable of hearing it themselves. Yet it is repeated over and over, like some wisdom that falls on deaf ears. The patient knows whether they are capable of healing. It is revealed in the first minutes of a consultation, in between the words of information. It underlies form.

The hidden signs of illness are expressed through gestures and speech patterns, whether the patient sits near or apart, looks into your eyes, or begins to cry uncontrollably on telling of their grief. This is what is calling to be healed. The body is a reflection of the inner state. The hormones shift to express that state. We are divided between attempting to address the stated problem and that which sustains it.

We must believe in ourselves. We must trust in our own ability to restore health and find solutions to problems as an inherent part of our survival and evolutionary resources. We need guidance in our health care, often more than one viewpoint. However, the vast entourage of medical and health practitioners promoting a complex array of methods can be overwhelming, confusing, and unpredictable.

It is not a question of one system versus another. To set one set of beliefs against another only leads to valuable resources wasted in conflict. Nor is it a matter of incorporating diverse information from different systems, as a complementary system. This tends to lead to the acceptance of the lowest common denominator in practice. Holistic shouldn't mean that the practitioner dabbles in every system, nor combines them. I am most skeptical of the person who says they practice several world systems, which individually take a lifetime of commitment to master. At its worst, Eclecticism represents the jack of all trades and the master of none.

The goal must be to provide the most suitable and appropriate care. Therefore we must incorporate a diverse range of expertise in respective fields. We must define what is competency in these fields, raising the standards of training to the level at which different schools of medicine and healing can coexist in an atmosphere of mutual respect.

Each system and practitioner draws patients of like mind. The lack of cooperation among practitioners and the lack of triage or communication perpetuates the inability to find solutions to our most difficult health problems. We would like to believe in the consistency of medicine, but even in the best hands, the lack of agreement even within a singular system can deteriorate our trust.

The Myths of Healing

Faith remains the mysterium of healing. Faith and prayer have proven to be one of the most successfully studied alternative healing practices. Yet faith must be generated from more than the dependence on an individual outside of ourselves. Faith must be enacted from a greater sphere than our personal lives. It is a connection with the Divine. We must expect from our practitioner skillfulness in therapeutics and a good sense of judgment without giving them sole authority. The innate intelligence of our bodies is the inner healer and must be called upon, by medicines, touch, awareness, and belief.

While practitioners defend their own methods with a mythological zeal, with statistics and philosophies that embellish their faith, ultimately we are individuals faced with the reality of our own suffering. Statistics may diagram the percentages of those who have recovered, but which group do we fall into, and at what cost? The studies themselves are frequently biased by the limitation of research to projects that will produce profitable outcomes.

Statistics are the attempt to isolate causative factors rather than an integrative approach. This is the foundation of a reductionist science. The method of deductive science is to maintain the limits for reproducibility. Nothing must be left to what we can't understand. It leaves nothing to contribute to medicine other than our medications. More importantly, it ignores the direct effects of such a singular approach. If the cure of pathology is solely the disappearance of symptoms, what is the pathogenesis of disease and what is the impact of a treatment on the overall ability of the organism to remain healthy? When we talk of suppression or cure it is not to exclude reductionist methods, but to expand our knowledge of their place in a more dynamic dimension.

Of course, the average patient is mainly concerned about their sinusitis, or some other common complaint. Their interest is in the disease to be treated. We have learned to focus on the presenting disease as if we had been attacked from the outside by malevolent germs and viruses. We identify with our diseases as if they were an inherent part of our being. We expect the disease should go away by taking medicine.

This expectation goes back to antiquity. The Egyptian Ebers Papyrus contained a long list of diseases distinguished by whether they could be cured or not. It is the same now. When I began my studies in botanical medicine I was dismayed by the long lists of herbs under a disease title. Which one was effective? What was the dosage? What were the distinguishing indications for one herb over another? I found that orthodox medicine was not as scientific in its treatment methods as it presented itself either. The arguments and dialogues which honed these systems still focused on their effects on a singular disease, as if they were something separate from the patient.

It is important to understand that it is not just the responsibility for a health care provider to eliminate a single problem. The practitioner should provide an overall plan for maintaining health. Health and disease are too important to be treated as distractions until the whole system collapses.

Health care professionals offer you their skill in their particular way of looking at the situation. In treating the context of disease, it would not be possible to know the potential for recovery without understanding the individual situation. It is not a statistical situation, but a life history that is to be treated.

Anything else remains either the recitation of anecdotal cases or symptoms of diseases cured by medicines, which looks no further than the evaluation of isolated events that we use to limit the definition of disease.

Reductionist treatment does not question how one disease relates to the other. It does not seek to know whether the elimination of symptoms may lead to a weakening of the immune system or a latent depression. It ignores a matrix of relationship.

We still carry ancient myths of healing with us. The white gown in the hospital was originally used by the Greeks in the Asclepian temples to remove the distinctions of class, so that a slave would receive treatment equal to that of an aristocrat. Priests who had special abilities to perceive the nature of disease were in attendance. Dreams were interpreted. The lines of the face or hands, the sound of voices, odor, vasculature, the color of skin, and discharges all told about the internal processes of diseases in the way the interpretation of the glyphs on an x-ray do today.

These primary sources of diagnosis should still be the central methodologies of the skilled physician. As critical as clinical laboratory methods are in their contribution to diagnosis, they are a confirmation of our ability to understand disease from history and physical examination, not a replacement. Looking at a computer readout does not tell us who we are dealing with and why. The descriptive method of disease and its natural history, found in century old medical books, can still help us understand how disease progresses, what are its subtleties of expression, and what peripheral processes may be involved. These old methods sought not so much to interpret observations as to simply record their relationships. It is unfortunate that the training in perception and physical diagnostic methods that was once the domain of every physician has now been relegated to the authority of the specialist.

In physics, Neils Bohr's concept of complementarity directed our attention to the significance of the observer's interaction with his subject. He determined in studying elementary particles of atoms that the perception of the observer infects the probable outcome in an experiment. The behavior of particles is a limited area of study. Bohr himself applied his concepts to diverse areas, including sociology and politics. These observations in physics may correspond, though, to any studies with unpredictable and random influences that influence their objectivity. The biases we establish as research methodology can affect our outcomes. Even our presence in the laboratory and clinic affects the results.

In healing, our lives are the experiment and our bodies the crucible. Unconscious ideas remain latent in both the formation of disease and in its interpretation. Whenever we are presented with a mystery our unconscious is constellated. Though we may attempt to explain disease by reducing them to a mechanism, we cannot ignore their implications and systemic effects. Even the word *syndrome* reveals that the order of disease is a complex, which when addressed as a singular element ignores the full effect of the disorder.

The Myths of Disease

An example of the unconscious archetypal influences on medical theory arose in the 1980s when science was confronted with the epidemic of AIDS. One of the theories proposed by early AIDS researchers suggested the disease originated in Haiti. This was not the first incidence of Haiti being the source for psychological projections when faced with an epidemic venereal disease. It reflected back to the sixteenth century when the epidemics of syphilis led to the introduction of Guiacum, a plant from Haiti, where the disease was believed to have come from. It was thought that the disease and the cure would come from the same place.

The importing of Guiacum brought great financial rewards to the ruling merchant class, the Fugers, but contributed little to the eradication of syphilis. The need to import foreign plants was fought by the great medical reformer, Theophrastus Bombastus von Hohenheim, known as Paracelsus (1493–1541). He proposed that medicines could be found within the local region,

[14]

if only their properties could be determined. He introduced the use of minerals, metals, and chemical salts into medicine. He stated that every substance was a medicine or a poison, depending on its dose and appropriate use. Paracelsus recommended minute doses of mercury for the treatment for syphilis. His criticism of Guiacum use and his descriptions of mercury toxicity stood in direct opposition to the commercial interests of his day. In 1529, Paracelsus published the first of what was to be eight books on the "French disease." He was censored by a decree based on the opinion of the Leipzig Medical Faculty and forced to leave Nuremberg and discontinue publishing his tracts on syphilis.

Today we would seem ignorant to suggest mercury as a medicine. The photographs of Eugene Smith show the disfiguring human effects of mercury poisoning in Minimata, Japan and Sabastio Salgado's depictions of the Brazilian gold mines where miners' exposure to mercury was commonplace as it leaked into the water systems and spread downstream. Up until the nineteenth century mercury was one of the most common pharmaceuticals. It was thought that the salivation produced by mercury was a detoxification process and that it purged the liver. Mercury was used in the lining of hats—thus the "Mad Hatter." It was used to preserve corpses for dissection by medical students. Mercury is indeed a powerful tool; it was used in the treatment of syphilis. Its toxicology reflects the pathology of syphilis in that mercury is stored in the fat of the central nervous system in an insidious, destructive manner. It is still used in homeopathy, commonly for childhood ear infections and neurological disorders.

Four hundred years after the first speculation of the origins of syphilis in Haiti, the same misinterpretation was projected. We can see the limitations of our own beliefs in our capacity for objectivity here. Although we strive for objectivity, the unconscious archetypal beliefs constellated during the outbreak of epidemics have generated similar fears and mistaken conclusions over the centuries. These fears of epidemics are not unwarranted. The Spanish flu of 1919 killed more people than World War I. It is these fears that often distract our attention from finding

[15]

solutions. We still contain our primitive behavior in light of our progress.

We have indeed progressed. The AIDS situation also speaks to our ability to use science to overcome these erroneous beliefs. The rather rapid discovery of the HIV virus provided a major tool for limiting its spread. There is no evidence that earlier systems of medicine were more capable with dealing with the destructive capacity of most epidemic diseases.

The Myths of Chemistry

Today our society has accepting the ruling myth of chemistry. The emerging dominance of isolated chemicals in medicine has never been solely a matter of scientific proof. The growth of chemical medicine occurred after World War II largely due to the efficacy of antibiotics. Until the 1940s botanical medicines were still an active part of the U.S. Pharmacopea. No double blind studies were ever conducted to compare the efficacy of a plant to its chemical analogue. The argument that isolating an active agent and synthesizing it would establish its consistency in dosage simply doesn't survive scrutiny. Many more complications occur from the so-called side effects that result when a singular physiological action is pushed than from the diverse interactions that occur naturally in plants and other biological substances. Certainly, any argument that considers plant medicine to be unsafe has to compare the isolated occurrences of poisoning from plants with the overwhelming commonality of poisoning from both over-the-counter and prescription medications.

Orthodox medicine evolved through the funding of lobbyists who could maintain the certainty of the patenting process. The paradigm of research was diminished to the size and perspective that could maintain this narrow process. We have established an economic oligarchy rather than a true scientific process. The social importance we attribute to medicine tends to obfuscate the influence of the medical industry on medical education and political decision making.

We are faced with the same crisis that led to the elimination of natural therapeutics from the training of physicians at the turn of the twentieth century. When one system dominates our understanding of life, it ignores the full potential for solving problems that may be available to us.

In the nineteenth century, several schools of medicine competed under the medical degree. The first national organization of physicians in the U.S. was the American Institute of Homeopathy founded in 1843. The American Medical Association was formed two years later to counteract the rise and success of homeopathy. At the time the medicine represented by the AMA was considered questionable, due to the physicians' prescriptions of medicines with deleterious and toxic side effects. Surgery was used to replace the inability to find adequate treatments in many cases. It was a primitive and crude period in the history of medicine.

By the 1880s, the patent pharmaceutical industry arose, making fortunes from the sales of three primary drugs, opium, cocaine, and calomel, a mercury preparation. This formed the financial basis for the support of an organization that would uphold the authority of the pharmaceutical companies to define the course of medicine. That organization was the American Medical Association. Prior to the pharmaceutical support of the AMA lobbying efforts and its journals and schools, the AMA was not a very effective political organization. It rapidly assumed dominance in the most influential political decisions concerning medical education and its practice in the twentieth century.

The battle among the different schools of medicine culminated with the Flexnor Report in 1913, which was influenced by the AMA and the need for the pharmaceutical industry to assure that patentable medicines would be taught in medical schools as the sole proponents of scientific medicine. This report, in fact, was influential in Congress, which used it as a standard in evaluating medical schools for accreditation and funding. As a result much of the diversity of thought in medicine was quickly eliminated.

Despite all our hopes in medical science, much is lost or ignored in the wealth of information that is available to the medical community. Useful research has come from Third World and Eastern European institutions, most of which is considered inadequate simply because of their origins. The studies would require repetition in a Western industrialized university setting to be accepted.

While the scientific method of critical thinking has raised the standard of evaluating treatment efficacy, it has also raised the cost prohibitively, so that research is now governed by a profit motive.

Unfortunately, the great questions of life and healing do not always fit the limitations of current science. This is why so many fundamental questions about chronic disease remain unanswered. Scientific inquiry is often founded on doubt, and it has always been the creative inquirer that has inspired us to look further than our current thought.

We are now in a critical period, as environmental and public health conditions have created the need for greater populations to survive together. The great forces that have been unleashed in the past century call on us to develop the wisdom to apply our new discoveries intelligently. The insights of chemists and physicists in the early part of this century demonstrated greater capabilities than their application in environmental poison and nuclear proliferation. Science has been both a behemoth of modern society and its salvation.

[18]

The Myths of Science

There is little exchange of information between the revolutions that are occurring in different fields of science. Discoveries in physics may not necessarily filter down to the biological sciences or be applied to medicine. Each school of science maintains its own interests. Biology is concerned with the genesis and transformation of the living physical form, while physics is concerned with the energetics of inanimate forms. They represent separate languages describing different dimensions in the same matrix. Yet biology is still deeply influenced by the field of physics, and new models are emerging that confirm the more generalized perspective of previous sciences. Molecular biology currently dominates funding of research to the disadvantage of any other specialties in science. But scientific paradigms are the shifting sands of truth, and what is believed today becomes the dogma of ignorance tomorrow. Too often physicians confuse their art with science. They state without doubt what they cannot defend. The angry cry of "nonsense" really means that it makes no sense to them. It remains outside their sphere of knowledge. To remain unaware of a wider point of view that is clearly described in current literature is ignorance. It is literally ignoring.

We need to create forums for dialogue, as each separate discipline tends to isolate itself in groups that agree with each other. Science and medicine can become a Tower of Babel, where each discussion feeds to perpetuate its own discipline, without questioning its weaknesses. The bastions of education and research become a hierarchy of competition rather than a collective search for truth. What deters the solutions sought remains evasive. The result is a language generated that communicates only to its adherents. In every clinical case there exists simpler and more elegant solutions than are usually applied. We need a forum for interspecies communication.

The alternative health care community is just as guilty in forming unsupportable belief and defenses. There is often an aversion to critical thinking, as if this would invalidate the foundations of their personal experience. Often diagnoses in alternative medicine are based on diagnostic machines or systems that can't be or are not verified. So patients may remain under care being treated for a disease they don't have, or which are secondary to an underlying problem. Yeast infections are a common diagnosis whose proliferation is secondary to disruption of the intestinal flora or urinary tract primarily by the overuse of antibiotics.

We spend tremendous efforts solving medical problems, often in situations where treatment lies outside the realm of medications. Most of the information we receive on nutrition is provided through university agricultural and veterinary programs under the funding of the food industry. Nutrition remains a minimal aspect of medicine. The dairy and meat industry still fund educational programs in our schools. They lobby to define government dietary recommendations, despite clear evidence contrary to those recommendations. Dieticians in hospitals determine what is adequate nutrition for a recovering or compromised patient and it is ubiquitously no better than the cafeteria food.

We reproach the tobacco industry for what is an individual's choice to destroy their health, while the insidious effects of the chemical industry are often ignored. Obviously no other country could inflict from outside the range of sickness and death subjected upon American citizens through environmental contaminants. Biological warfare is being fought in our own country by our own industries. At what cost? What is the cost to our society of supporting such a fundamentally ignorant attitude towards preventive medicine?

We have gained a great understanding of the pathogenesis of disease in the past century. Yet the profoundest impact of modern medicine has not come necessarily from the realm of therapeutic agents, but from public health, sanitation, and nutrition. These ideas, when newly conceived, were not so readily accepted as we would think today. As recently as the early 1960s the notion that cigarette smoking was related to lung cancer was rejected by most medical societies.

The scientific establishment has a long history for ignoring the insights of progressive physicians and scientists. Rather than scientific inquiry, they sought inquisition. The most famous of these was the inquisition of Galileo, in which Church officials refused to look through his telescope because it would threaten to destroy the cosmological beliefs set forth in Church doctrine.

Ignaz Semelweiss was a nineteenth-century obstetrician who literally went mad trying to convince surgeons to wash their hands between deliveries and surgeries to prevent puerperal infections, the leading cause of death in women following childbirth. Semmelweiss found that the doctors would come directly from autopsies to examine women post delivery, thereby infecting them. He required physicians on the ward he supervised to scrub their hands and soak them in a chlorinated lime solution before and after entering the delivery ward. Within a few months, the obstetrical death rate dropped from eighteen percent to one and two tenths percent on his ward.

One might expect that this would have been enough to convince the medical community of the importance of sanitation. Instead, the Chief of Service, for reasons of personal antagonism, condemned Dr. Semmelweiss, arranged for having his rank lowered, and limited his practicing privileges. Semelweiss's report to the Medical Society was denounced and his subsequent book that he wrote ten years after his initial discoveries went unnoticed, denounced even by the scientist Virchow. Eventually his life ended tragically. His failure to convince his colleagues led to his eventual institutionalization in a mental asylum. He died tragically from the same original insight that led him to his discoveries, an infection following a finger cut during surgery.

It was not until the work of Joseph Lister (despite initially being discredited by the medical societies) found its way into the surgical practices of Parisian hospitals that an understanding of the dangers of infections came to be respected. Lister proposed the use of carbonic acid in the disinfection of open wounds. These ideas followed the work of Pasteur, who introduced sterilization by boiling. Obviously, boiling was not appropriate in living human tissue. The practicing physicians of the time treated the ideas of Pasteur and his colleagues on the relationship between bacteria and infections with disregard and hostility.

While the development of specific antibiotics for pathological agents profoundly improved success in treating infectious disease, a hidden cost has emerged. The overuse of antibiotics to treat common ailments has led to a disruption of the internal microbiological ecosystems in our bodies. Antibiotics affect not only the bacteria we wish to eliminate, but destroy the beneficial flora which maintain the internal balance of bacterial growth. A bacterium such as Staphylococcus can be pathological, but also normal bacteria that are normally maintained in balance can overgrow and become pathological under antibiotic treatment. This problem has been recognized by some medical authors, such as Boyd, who states in his *Textbook of*

Medicine, "We recognize that the pattern of disease has changed out of recognition during the last thirty to forty years owing to modern drugs, particularly the antibiotics."

The bacterial flora that lines our gut is one of the primary boundaries of the immune system. It prevents foreign agents from entering the bloodstream through the gut. The abuse of antibiotics is a contributing factor to the modern prevalence of childhood allergies.

The balance of intestinal bacterial flora was the central idea in the work of Elie Metchnikoff (1845–1916), a contemporary of Pasteur's and a researcher at the Pasteur Institute, who challenged the focus on bacteria as the central cause of disease. Metchnikoff was one of the early discoverers of cellular immunity, which is the ability of the immune system to fight off disease. He believed the basis for disease to be the susceptibility of the organism, originating in the disruption of the internal bacterial environment. He saw disease as a disturbance of the terrain or soil of the body, rather than the influence solely of the infectious agent. Like a seed implanted upon fertile soil, the disease was the result of environmental conditions. Metchnikoff introduced the use of yogurt and lactobacillus cultures as preventative measures to strengthen the gut flora.

Edward Bach (1886–1936), a London homeopath and gastroenterologist who is remembered mostly for his development of the Bach flower remedies, in fact spent much of his career studying and developing the use of bacterial flora as medicines in treating chronic diseases. It was not until he retired that he began his study of the use of flower essences.

The current overuse of antibiotics in orthodox medicine has not developed from the initial discoveries that led to the favorable and appropriate use of antibiotics in life-threatening infections. It has arisen from a similar conceptual framework that led to the rise of pesticides and the chemical industry as the salvation of farmers, and at the same cost. The mechanical approach to the elimination of unwanted organisms ignores the conditions which lead to their proliferation. In medicine and agriculture, it is the underlying susceptibilities of the organism or field, the diseased state, which permits the overgrowth of a pathogen. Many of the organisms that are designated as pathogens occur naturally or are ubiquitous in the environment. When an imbalance occurs due to lack of appropriate nutrition, defects in the immune response, or debilitating influences, such as environmental conditions or emotional stress (and it is proposed by some that plants have their own problems to deal with), the system becomes vulnerable. This vulnerability may lead to a disruption in the bacterial environment and a subsequent overgrowth of the infectious organism.

Think of a field or a meadow. In their natural states, many plants coexist in the natural development of an ecosystem. When man decides to remove certain unsightly plants that are seen as weeds, suddenly greater and greater energy is required to maintain this new unintegrated system. Look at our lawns, how much water and fertilizer are required. Biological systems thrive on diversity. When we do not cultivate the widely adapted, naturally occurring species of vegetation in favor of hybrids, we may simplify our ability to harvest by means of mass production. However, a monoculture is more susceptible to disease. This creates reliance not only on seed companies, because hybrids are unable to produce seed for next year's crop, but also on pesticides which become necessary to support the inadequate defenses of an artificial system.

We are seeds and our development depends on the soil of our lives. Medicines act often to make us the same, to control behavior or symptoms. It seeks the norm rather than the diverse. In its ultimate guise, medicine becomes the work of dermatologists and plastic surgeons, where surface anatomy must conform to the expectations of magazines.

[23]

ALLOPATHY: THE MYTHS OF MODERN MEDICINE

The use of drugs as an antagonist to disease is the definition for an allopathic approach. The word *allopathic* comes from the Greek, meaning contrary to disease. It represents the culmination of mechanistic theory in medicine and represents the underlying theory of orthodox practice. Often symptoms and diseases are seen as unrelated. The appearance of a disease is not often seen as related to previous diseases in the individual's history. In homeopathic theory the results of allopathic treatment can lead to suppression. The suppressive results that can pervade this method often lead to a deeper and more internal disorganization. This is expressed through the side effects of medications, or even more seriously in subsequent disorders that are treated separately, as their relationship is ignored. There are no side effects, only direct effects taken out of context.

Although medicines can act to alter a disease process that has rapidly progressed, they don't necessarily address the ground of its development. That is why it is so important to understand the nature of disease and the interrelationship of its manifestations. Much of what is treated symptomatically as an acute or temporary problem is in fact an expression of our chronic problem, which therefore returns for a repeated treatment. An acute disease is a temporary, self-limiting condition usually not experienced previously. It is usually collective, a contagion that has passed from one individual or environment to others. This might be a flu, a sudden infection, a reaction to contaminated food, or something similar. There can be a chronic influence to a flu, but it would most likely be found in the psychology of the group. Bad news, economic predictions, etcetera, can bring on a widespread weakening of the immune system. When the media plays up disasters, our bodies react as well.

Problems such as repeated ear infections, strep throats, allergies, and herpes outbreaks are not acute diseases but acute manifestations of the underlying chronic condition that must be treated as such. Even our susceptibility to infections is a result of our chronic state.

The body doesn't heal with big guns and magic bullets. It is more like a quail in the woods whispering to its mate, reminding it of something it has forgotten or of danger it has ignored. Healing doesn't come from the medicine itself. It comes from the ability of the medicine to call attention to a self-destructive disturbance. It is an internal self-regulating process. If we see disease from a mechanical perspective, we face the task of eliminating it. However, if we see disease as a part of our being, our beingness, then it must be touched by healing rather than manipulated by force.

We believe in the intelligence of the body that God has created. We have evolved with remarkable sophistication. As an organism we are capable of deep inherent knowledge and a capacity for healing. The potentials of the body and psyche are greater than the mind of the physician. Therefore, it is our duty to respect the natural laws that govern this tremendous act of creation. If these laws are ignored, chaos results. If we do not see how symptoms fit into the greater scheme of our lives at the onset of illness, we miss the opportunity to understand their function and resolution. So if we treat a symptom as an acute problem that we wish to eliminate, we may actually be ridding ourselves of the only clues for healing that the body is capable of giving us. It is like destroying evidence in a murder case because we are not capable of understanding its use. If the origins of disease are not addressed, the messages become disrupted or silenced. Disease is often described as a metaphor for war, and viewed as an enemy to be destroyed rather than a purposeful, intelligent response of the organism. The use of force ignores the body's abilities to receive messages through enemy lines. We have built defenses throughout our lives that represent a greater effort than that undertaken by a samurai or special forces agent, and have utilized tremendous energy in their creation.

When force is used, the natural responses are resistance and further defense. Our natural defense systems are more sophisticated and powerful than we acknowledge, but we undermine them with therapeutic applications that overwhelm these resources. We must send selective messages that induce a specific response, a hypnotic suggestion that reeducates our system rather than attempting to dominate it. The remedy is a diplomat, not a warrior. Perhaps this means we need a peace movement within our bodies and minds.

Is this always the case? Probably not. There is a time when it is best to act decisively in eradicating a problem. But we must understand what we are dealing with. It is not often an act of fate, an event from outside. This is not just our disease; it is our history; it is our bodies and our selves.

It is hard not to isolate one stage of the process grasping for an explanation. If each manifestation of disease is treated separately, then no opportunity exists to engage the body's inherent defenses. The longer the message is disrupted, the more difficult it becomes to hear it, and the body's ability to recover becomes diminished.

In response to many diseases the normal and pathological responses of the cell are so closely interrelated that only the body's own self-regulating mechanisms can have an effect. Any treatment which disturbs these mechanisms rather than engaging them can disrupt this vital intelligence of the body.

I don't believe we can generalize why a person is sick. To maintain that anyone has created their own disease is a malicious attitude. It ignores our understanding of the unconscious and its ability to understand what our capacity is at the moment. It forgets the weak links in the chain of our ancestral inheritance, the latent expressions of viral agents and the genetic code. It is an unforgiving attitude toward our bodies and their limitations. If we accept that the cause of disease is not linear and that mechanisms, whether physiological or psychological, are interrelated, then we cannot accept a singular causality. The cause of disease cannot be known.

We begin to see the terrain or soil, which allows the conditions for disease to arise, maintains it, and allows its proliferation. Disease may be interpreted from various facets, yet the disease arises from within. We may agree on a diagnosis of infection, which began during a depression, which elicited a period of weakened immunity, whose origins could be a grief experienced, which related to an early childhood experience, and ad infinitum. In other words, disease can be interpreted on any level. What is important is understanding at which level it is to be addressed. The treatment reflects the depth of understanding of the situation, and the depth of skill and understanding of the method that is utilized. The rule of thumb is the more medicines used the less specificity is possible. The more peripheral the treatment, the more complex the approach. The more cen-

[26]

tral the treatment, the simpler the approach until ultimately there is only one medicine.

Life is not as linear as we would like to structure it. As in a dream, our memories try to place events in a coherent fashion so that we can comprehend our world. When we struggle to achieve a plateau, greater peaks rise into our view. We long for a quiescent moment, yet it is the challenges that stimulate our growth.

Disease is such a challenge. It is an expression of how we must face our challenges. It is not some goal we have set for ourselves through our will to achieve, but the demand that we face who we are. The most common cause of illness is the split between who we are and who we think we should be. It is the inability to find acceptance from ourselves and others, to allow grace into our lives. It is our will attempting to define our world rather than finding our place in it.

Chapter Two

Oп the Importaпce of Apprenticeship: The Renaissance of Natural Medicine

The renaissance of natural medicines was generated from the environmental politic. It was formed from the roots of natural philosophy. Somehow we knew there was a medicine that lay hidden in the earth, that wasn't produced by the rise of large chemical industries. There was more that was sought. The lost traditions that were handed down from generation to generation were the ground for our immersion. We modeled ourselves on the guilds, scholars, mystics, and elders who gave their knowledge through personal transmission and guidance. Quietly, outside the university, was a tradition that spoke directly, without the walls of specialization. We sought a myth, a science passed by or lost, a system, or an experience that would reveal the wisdom of the past.

I wanted to know if the old books were true, or were they ignorance and metaphor. Was there forgotten truths hidden in untranslatable languages or mistaken concepts? Were the old American Indian herbalists just poking fun at young inquisitive anthropologists, or was there something substantial there? Was there a medicine even more substantial than what we use today?

I began at a Quaker boarding school. My friend had been given the book, *American Indian Medicine,* by Virgil Vogel. It lay on his pillow like it was an altar. We went into the woods to find the plants. There we found Jack in the pulpit *(Arum triphyllum),* Skunk cabbage *(Symplocarpus foetidus),* Skullcap *(Scutellaria lateriflora),* Joe Pye Weed *(Eupatorium purpureum),* and Boneset *(Eupatorium perfoliatum).* We poisoned ourselves to find if the descriptions of the plant effects were accurate. Jack in the pulpit made our throats dry and raw. We relished the acrid tastes, the pungent aromas, minerals of roots and leaves, and the beauty of the flowers. And we formed from these trials our re-experience of the dialogue between native and pioneer, plant and sensory investigator. We felt the strength of the plants, their ability to change the balance of our bodies.

By my senior year in high school, I had entered into a full study of botanicals. I took a course in the basement of a bookstore that served as an herb shop. It was there that I heard mentioned that a nearby hospital had been a homeopathic hospital. I found that a homeopathic pharmacy still existed in the basement and that two old surgeons still used it in their practices.

I didn't even know what the word meant, but it held my attention. They mentioned a Flower Homeopathic Hospital that had existed in New York City, and my imagination was triggered. What would it mean to use flowers as medicine? How could a hospital manage severe illness with such simple tools? It was not until twenty years later that I found out the Flower Hospital in New York had been named after the Flower family. But I was not entirely mistaken. Flowers were the source of many of our most significant medicines. They represent our most complex chemical messengers. Like pheromones, perfumes, and fancy clothes, they are an expression in the plant world like our own selves showing off and attracting our mates.

Finding my Teachers

I sought apprenticeship after a long term of study. I had met people who practiced solely after having read books, but they did not have the experience or the demonstrable results to convince me of their knowledge. They too were still seeking, trying to figure out what was there. I corresponded with doctors in England and Greece trying to find the threads that would lead to a true education. I didn't want to mimic or recite from books; I wanted to know from conviction. There was no direct way. Many of the great teachers had spent years struggling to keep the traditions alive without much support or respect from their colleagues. Their meetings were poorly attended. In the U.S. they maintained isolated practices, where few came to study.

While I was attending college, I continued my herbal studies in Vermont with a wonderful woman, Adele Dawson. Adele lived in the next town, Marshfield. Entering Marshfield, the sign said "Welcome to Mars"—since someone had painted over the "hfield". Adele had her house and barn at the base of one of Vermont's largest waterfalls. She had a remarkable garden of flowers and vegetables covering the whole hill beside it. Adele was an artist and the barn was her studio. Her house was a constant gathering place for her students, with regular meetings and yearly herb festivals.

Adele would teach by just having us join in her life, preparing food and herbs, or just reading and talking. She was a lover of life. She was short and wiry. Her back was hunched over. She rode old jalopies down the steep slope from her house, and in the winter she would often have fender benders or worse. She would just laugh it off saying the car wasn't worth anything anyway.

She never showed off her knowledge, but if you looked in her library, there was always a wealth of books to inspire conversation. Like most good herbalists, she spoke to the plants and fairies. She would tell the insects they would have to leave a certain area of the garden or she would be forced to take measures, and they usually cooperated.

Soon I found an article. It was called "Why I am a Homeopath" by Allan Sutherland, M.D. of Brattleboro, Vermont. I was impressed by his story, so I found his number and phoned him. Though he was pleasant and rather surprised at my call, it was not a good time for me to visit him. His wife was dying at the time and he was engaged in taking care of her.

The next year I traveled to the West Coast. I applied for a job as a baker at a Tibetan Buddhist monastery run by Tarthung Tulku, who had the wisdom to suggest to me that I not get so involved in one place, but to experience all that the Bay Area had to offer. So I began by studying many methods of healing. I bought books in Berkeley, juiced wheatgrass, and did yoga everyday. There was a jazz and salsa group that practiced in the house. I took a few classes and attended lectures and poetry readings.

I became involved in an institute that worked on the development of intuition. But I felt I didn't have the emotional development to work with others on an inner level yet. And I used my understanding of medicines to distance myself from any concept of my personal involvement in healing. At age eighteen my boundaries were too acute.

I left Berkeley and hitchhiked through the Northwest. I was picked up by a family whose aching van barely made it through the mountainous terrain. We passed a rock formation they were convinced was the face of an Indian. The car died. We were stranded and found a place near the road to camp. It was a year since I had called Dr. Sutherland. That night I dreamed that this family's baby had a rash on its face, and I knew it was the resolution of something deeper that had passed from the mother to the child. I knew that if it were treated as a superficial problem, it would never be resolved. It was an opportunity. I told them to call Dr. Sutherland.

When I awoke, I found a public phone and called him. His wife had passed away since we had last talked and he invited me to visit his clinic. I didn't know that for the past twenty-five years Dr. Sutherland had been the Dean of the only postgraduate course in homeopathy in the U.S. I didn't know that he was the last editor of the *Homeopathic Recorder,* which chronicled the guild of classical homeopaths in the United States.

I trusted my dream. I believed in the fabric of some archaic web I was caught up in. It was like some Biblical vision which no one believed anymore, some minor prophecy that had lost its meaning in the modern world. And being young, I was a bit of a fanatic.

I crossed the country. I rode with a troupe of traveling wrestling midgets through Montana. I read lectures on *Materia Medica,* which described the clinical uses of medicines, and a mysterious text on alchemy. They suited each other, the somber, tedious, descriptive, turn-of-the-century homeopathic discourse and the symbolic philosophical chemistry of Europe and Ancient Egypt. I carried herbs in plastic bags and homeopathic medicines in vials, treating people with my raw knowledge. This was my journey back to the Eastern part of the country. The West Coast was syncretic, synthesizing, and initiating broad ranges of thought. The East had maintained a purity of tradition.

I got a job working at a nursing home, taking care of the dying and the elderly who had been cast aside. I stayed with Dr. Sutherland initially, in a room with his son's old school banners still on the walls. His late wife's vanity was left untouched in his bedroom, though he had grown a goatee since her death which she would have disapproved of.

I read his books, at least the half that were medical; the others were mostly history books, primarily on the Civil War. Soon I found a place to live on a farm in Putney, the next town north. I sat in at the Green Mountain Health Clinic on the days Dr. Sutherland treated patients and studied his cases at night, analyzing and differentiating which medicines would be appropriate and which ones I would have chosen. The next day we would review my choices before the patients came.

He gave me books; An 1892 copy of *A Textbook of Materia Medica and Therapeutics,* by Cowperthwaite, Boenninghausen's *Therapeutic Pocketbook* with annotations handwritten by his teacher, Herbert Roberts, and *Repertory of the Homeopathic Materia Medica,* by James Tyler Kent that had been given to him by Dr. Elizabeth Wright-Hubbard.

I began to see that common diseases that were considered

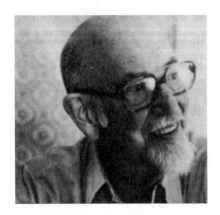

Allan Sutherland, M.D.

incurable were resolved through understanding what characterized their individuality. Then the mass of information began to take form. Each disease and medicine had many representations. It was a matter of perceiving their relationship, like seeing someone you know in a crowd. It was a sense of recognition which developed slowly, gradually finding the key that fit. I was trying to fit into the role of someone who knew, though I was young, fumbling, and struggling. Dr. Sutherland would kid me about my diet. He'd look in the pot and ask me what kind of grass I was eating. He would smoke in front of patients. He could pull that gruff Vermont, New England orneriness, as well as be jovial and kind.

We traveled that summer to Millersville, Pennsylvania where the only American post-graduate program in homeopathy was conducted.

I assumed he was eternal, but I was wrong. He sent me back to school to get my pre-medical studies under my belt, and in January I got a letter from his son that he had passed. He had called a cab to take him to the hospital, where he had worked since it was built. He just asked for a bed and before there was a chance for him to be examined he was gone. I was shocked. He was so vital that I never thought he would die so soon. I felt guilty for having returned to school. For me, my teachers were the grandparents I never had, as they had died before I was born.

I was lost for where to go from there. I benefited from the kindness of Edward Whitmont, a Jungian psychiatrist and homeopath who I had visited at his homes in Vermont and in New York. He gave of his time and advice freely and helped me keep to my path. I thought I would pursue further training in Jungian psychology with him, but he fortunately pointed out I had enough to do.

The summer before Dr. Sutherland had passed he mentioned a reclusive homeopath who practiced in Michigan, and suggested I visit her. I had heard of her when we were in Millersville;

she had the reputation of a legendary practitioner. They said she never took appointments as she no longer had a phone, but she saw patients who came to her door long into the night.

I knew I had to meet her.

I somehow found the directions to Rood's Lake Road outside of Lapeer, Michigan. Down past the raceway where they held drag races on Sundays, the road turned to dirt. Not far on the left was a small white farmhouse where Dr. Rood saw her patients.

When I arrived, patients had lined themselves in her driveway and on the front porch, picnicking and talking among themselves, waiting for their turn to see this mysterious doctor. I sat with them as they told me the stories of her cures of their families and friends, until finally Dr. Rood appeared at the side door to feed the growing family of cats waiting there for her.

I walked over and introduced myself. I told her I had worked with Dr. Sutherland, whom I knew she had known. "Oh, Dr. Sutherland," she exclaimed, "I love him." Then she discretely added, "professionally, of course." Dr. Rood had never been married. She told me her mother had encouraged her to read books. But to her mother's chagrin, she became so engrossed with books that she had no time for her brother's friends who came by to visit. She attended the University of Michigan and was the sole woman in her graduate physics program. She then went to New York Homeopathic Medical College and lived in New York City. When I told her I had come to learn from her, she told me to wait outside under a tree till she had some time to talk.

I waited for what seemed like hours. Slowly the clouds above got darker and a storm began approaching from the west. I felt a few large drops of rain as Dr. Rood appeared at the side door again and shouted, "you better come in." I sat in the corner of her living room in a rocking chair. Her living room was crowded. It was lined with bookshelves, medicine chests, dogs and cats, piles of books, clean dishes, fruit and bread baskets covered with linen napkins, and of course whole families of patients discussing their problems, or just nodding in agreement at Dr. Rood. This was not a normal physician's office; Dr. Rood worked with a kitchen apron on.

As a physicist who had worked in the 1920s on the early quantum theories, she was always pursuing the most recent knowledge in medicine and science. Her desks contained the most recent scientific journals. More importantly, she showed me how to read scientific literature in the context of homeopathic thought. She saw the connection between current insights and the past traditions and would demonstrate how basic scientific research could be applied clinically in homeopathic terms.

Dr. Rood had studied with Arthur Grimmer, a Chicago homeopath who had taken over James T. Kent's practice. She was one of the few left in the greatest lineages of homeopathy. Dr. Grimmer was renown for his work in cancer and the introduction of cadmium salts in its treatment. He was also influential in investigating the works of Albert Abrams, a San Francisco physician whose method of testing the body through abdominal percussion and neurological reflexes developed into the early practices of radionic instruments and kinesiology.

Earlier in her practice, Dr. Rood had built a Faraday cage out of copper wires in a room to remove the influence of external electrical forces. In her difficult cancer cases, she would assess samples of blood using the Abrams method in this room. When I asked her why she no longer used the Abrams method, she responded that she preferred working directly with the patients and that she had learned what she had needed from doing those experiments.

Her teaching style was definitely Socratic. When I would ask something, she would reply, "Oh you should think about that." Then maybe three days later she would be talking to a patient and go into a long discourse, answering my question. The patient, of course, would have no idea why she was telling them all the esoterics of science and medicine, but I got it. She would even turn the vial of medicine away from me so I had to figure out what she had given. It took me four years of visiting her before I could draw out of her some of her more remarkable secrets.

She had a large scab that persisted on her forehead between her eyebrows. Some thought it was actually a skin cancer, but it never grew. Her left cheekbone was collapsed from a surgery that resulted after a tooth infection spread. She had the quality that only a Jedi master could have. She was an eccentric who could exist freely in conservative subcultures of America. In fact, many times she reminded me of Yoda, the teacher in the Star Wars movies.

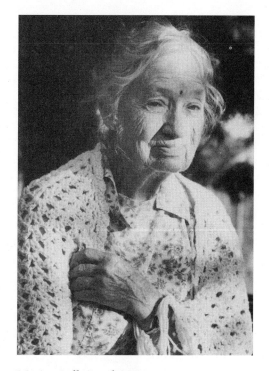

One night we had stayed up until three in the morning seeing patients. Finally when the last patient had left, I made some tea. As we sat together I asked her, "Dr. Rood, a lot of your patients say you're psychic, what does that mean to you?" I knew if I asked her directly she would never have answered such a question. But she just looked up and said, "You just don't talk about these things."

Marion Belle Rood, M.D.

Another time an impatient man left late at night before his turn. On looking out the porch door, Dr. Rood just exclaimed, "Oh, he must have felt so much better just sitting there he didn't need to stay!"

Whenever I would arrive each summer, she would modestly claim, "What are you doing here? I can't have you stay here. What would the neighbors think?" As if the neighbors were concerned about a man in his twenties staying with a woman in her eighties down the road. I had written her, telling her I would be coming, but the letter may still be sitting under some magazines. And the curious thing was that after each summer she always told me I was welcome to come back.

Those were my initiatory training days.

[37]

Chapter Three

HOMEOPATHY: A MODEL OF HOLISTIC THERAPEUTICS

*There are ways and places in which we touch each other
which are not known until long after the fact. A slow
acting potency as in medicine. We will never know fully
what the effect has been, or how it has changed us.
Even the awareness in retrospect is not fully awake to it.
Each time a principle of completion reaches us, the angle
of vision changes. We are never the same one as before.*

—Theodore Enslin

The search for healing has led mankind through diverse and
often conflicting methodologies. The history of medicine is an
abstract of this wide range of experiences, an interpretation,
often casting aside pearls of wisdom which did not fit into the
current paradigm of science.

Homeopathy is one of the most successful challenges to mechanistic methods in medicine. The homeopathic school of medicine was founded by Samuel Hahnemann (1755–1843), a German physician, in the late 1700s. Hahnemann challenged the attempts of physiologists to isolate disease processes as the sole cause of disease. He concluded that medicine could not be based on the shifting sands of medical theories, but must have a rational basis. He asserted that attempts to manipulate physiology with medications were insufficient, since they did not address the integrity and complexity of the organism as a whole. He stated that the mental and emotional symptoms of the sick were to be given priority in understanding the disease process, as well as those symptoms that characterize the uniqueness of the individual symptoms. The philosophy of homeopathy is: Treat the patient, not the disease.

Hahnemann had to confront the use of toxic medications and improper treatment of the sick. Having gained a reputation in analytical chemistry and medicine, and as a writer on public health, he recommended sanitation methods, which led to the prevention of infectious disease. He wrote against the mistreatment of the mentally ill, suggesting it was a treatable disease. Before his work on homeopathic medicines, he developed a soluble form of mercury and a safer method for its use. His treatise on arsenic poisoning is still considered authoritative.

However, he was discontented with his inability to treat patients successfully on a consistent basis and concluded that he was often doing them more harm than good. Retiring from practice in 1782, he spent the next fourteen years earning a meager living doing chemical research, writing and translating medical works from English, French, Italian, and Latin. About this decision, he wrote:

> It was painful for me to grope in the dark, guided only by books in the treatment of the sick. To prescribe according to this or that fanciful view of the nature of diseases, substances that owed to mere opinion their place in the *Materia Medica*. I had conscientious scruples about treating unknown morbid states in my fel-

Samuel Hahnemann

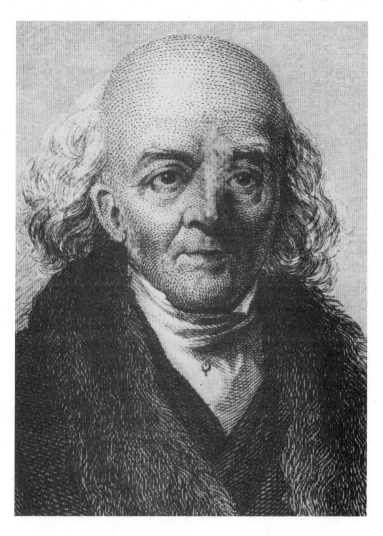

[41]

low suffering creatures with these unknown medicines which, being powerful substances, may if they were not exactly suitable (and how could the physician know whether they were suitable or not, seeing their peculiar special actions were not yet elucidated) easily change life into death, or produce new affections and chronic ailments, which are often more difficult to remove than the original disease.

—from the *Lesser Writings*

In 1790, during his translation of Scottish physician William Cullen he added a footnote disagreeing with Cullen's conclusions about cinchona bark, from which Quinine is derived. Cullen wrote that cinchona bark's effectiveness in malaria was due to its "bitter and astringent" qualities. Hahnemann, in a footnote to his translation, argued that there were several drugs in common usage that in smaller doses had greater bitter and astringent qualities, yet had no specific action upon fevers. As an experiment, Hahnemann took four drachms of cinchona twice daily, and soon developed the intermittent fevers common to malaria. Upon ceasing the drug, the symptoms disappeared.

THE LAW OF SIMILARS: LIKE TREATS LIKE

Hahnemann was not the first to test the effects of medicines on healthy persons to determine their range of curative action. However, he was unique in elucidating the importance of understanding the diversity of symptoms, both physical and mental, produced by the medicine as a descriptive representation of the psychosomatic syndromes they were capable of curing. Hahnemann defined his method of testing medicines on healthy people as "provings." He expanded his investigations to include a wide range of medicines, including botanical, animal, mineral, and chemical substances.

Recent medical literature has contained examples of inadvertent provings: In 1983, a study in the New England Journal of Medicine reported that pyridoxine (vitamin B_6), which is used in some types of peripheral neuropathies, is also capable of producing neuropathies when given in larger doses.

It is not by accident that disease arises. It functions to ward off deeper and more internal disorganization. Hahnemann's empirical investigations led not only to new applications of medicines, but provided a method for integrating the physical, mental, and emotional effects of a drug. This allowed for the treatment of the totality of the patient's symptoms as a dynamic pattern of interaction. Homeopathic treatment aims at stimulating the organism's inherent defense mechanisms. When medications are used solely for their physiological effect, they run the risk of creating dependency and disrupting vital immunological, hormonal, and emotional responses.

Considering the vitalistic perspective of the homeopathic approach, a clear definition of cure is necessary to establish the treatment goal. Since the patient's symptoms are viewed as the expression of the body's attempts to heal itself, any symptomatic treatment which masks the symptom at the cost of the overall vitality and function of the individual is considered negligent by the homeopathic practitioner. For example, if a child's eczema is treated and appears to resolve, but is followed by asthma, fatigue, and confusion it would not be considered accidental or unrelated. Cortisone, which is often used in these situations, is well known as an immunosuppressive anti-inflammatory. It is precisely these inflammatory responses that are common in eczema, asthma, and allergies. Therefore, under proper homeopathic treatment, the asthma is treated as a suppressed condition and an appropriate response would be an improvement of the asthma with a possible return of the eczema, followed by its subsequent alleviation.

HERING'S LAWS OF CURE

[43]

Constantine Hering, M.D. (1800–1880), is considered the Father of American Homeopathy, establishing the first homeopathic medical school and hospital in the United States in 1835. It later moved from its original site in Allentown, Pennsylvania to Philadelphia, where it remains today as an orthodox medical school: Hahnemann Medical College. Hering's promotion of homeopathy and the development of new medicines was equaled only by Hahnemann himself. His ten volume work, *The Guid-*

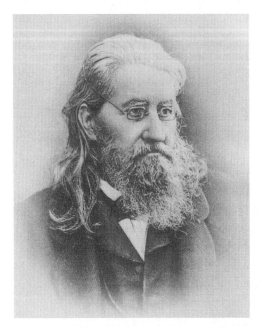

Constantine Hering

ing Symptoms of Our Materia Medica, remains a definitive work on clinical verifications of the homeopathic approach. Hering collected these confirmations as he conducted his rounds at the college hospital, in his private practice, and through correspondence. It is unfortunate that of the many medicines introduced by Hering, only nitroglycerin remains in orthodox practice as a tribute to his medical genius.

Hering described Hahnemann's observations in a set of guidelines for evaluating curative responses. These principles could be applied to any healing process, regardless of its methods. In true healing, according to these observations, symptoms will follow the following patterns:

- From above downward through the body to its extremities.
- From within to without, often in the form of discharges and other eliminative processes.
- From the most important organs to the least important organs. For example, the central nervous system or other life dependent systems would be seen as central, while the skin would be more peripheral.

And finally,

- In reverse order of their appearance, that is with the reappearance of symptoms unwinding an Ariadnian thread of pathological history.

Mental and emotional symptoms are most central in homeopathic theory. These symptoms are viewed as positive homeostatic mechanisms, demonstrating purposeful strategies to maintain balance. Neurotic symptoms are understood to be more functional than self-destructive and suicidal ideations. It is also noted that persons who have deep psychological disturbances do not manifest many acute ailments, such as flus. This is because the center of gravity of the patient's illness is at a deep level and therefore the defense mechanisms focus their energies on the most essential requirements for the individual's survival.

Furthermore, under successful treatment of disorders of a serious nature, patients do not always remember their previous symptoms.

Why is this? It would seem that the self-protective nature of the defense mechanisms of our psyche relieve our conscious memory of the state we have experienced. So a schizophrenic person, or even someone who has recovered from a physical shock or injury, does not needlessly continue to reexperience their suffering.

If disease states are produced and expressed unconsciously or subconsciously, then the treatment must be capable of reaching the level at which the disease is enacted.

The Law of Similars reminds the body and psyche of a situation which it has become unconscious of responding to. Like a virus which has entered the cell and is no longer recognized as foreign, yet still produces illness, we use the medicines to remind the organism of its presence. No matter how much we attempt to talk ourselves into getting well, we still respond in chronic patterns. Psychological models often rely on providing coping mechanisms, without the necessary integration of the problem. It is the self- regulating capacity of the psyche which grounds the problem most effectively. It is always giving us the clues for redeeming the situation if we are capable of hearing them.

Disease and cure must also be considered in the context of the culture and belief systems of the patient. Much of what we consider as disease arises from the individual's inability to find meaning and purpose, as well as emotional expression. Many forms of healing enable the person to integrate into the fabric of daily life and provide ways to help the person address personal needs for fulfillment.

The mind should be capable of functioning with clarity, rationality, coherence, and logical sequence. It should be capable of engaging in creative service for the good of others, as well

[45]

as for oneself, demonstrating a freedom from selfishness and possessiveness. On the emotional level, there should be a state of serenity free from being controlled by passion, a state that should not be confused with lack of emotional response generated as a protection against emotional vulnerability. To experience compassion means to feel with passion. It is a dynamic state, not just a quiescent one. It is human in its reality. Finally, on the physical level, there should be freedom from pain. The healing person should experience a subjective sense of well-being and a progressive increase in vitality.

HAHNEMANN'S DEFINITIONS OF ALLOPATHY

Hahnemann defined the application of medicines whose purpose was limited to altering physiology or acting as an antagonist to disease as the practice of "allopathy" (*allo* meaning contrary in Greek). In this method, diagnosis becomes the focus of practice. In medical practice today, much of prescribing is based on laboratory values rather than clinical diagnosis. Therefore, symptoms that are not confirmed by the diagnosis are considered unrelated. The pharmacological approach is often limited to the end results of disease rather than the origins of pathogenesis.

[46]

Since only the primary action of the pharmaceutical agent is utilized in treating a specific disease state, the remaining physiological as well as psychological effects are ignored or classified as side effects. Hahnemann demonstrated through clinical verification of his theories that medicines should have no side effects if they are applied with the understanding of their systemic action. In fact, many of the symptoms disregarded by pharmacologists as secondary to a medicine's principle action are homeopathic indications for the accuracy of its prescription.

It is precisely this synergism of effects that allows the homeopath to individualize his prescription. Hahnemann questioned the usefulness of testing drugs on animals. He observed that pigs could safely eat *Nux vomica* in quantities that would immediately kill humans. Dogs could eat *Aconite napellus* (monkshood), a deadly poison to humans, without injury. He also rejected testing the method of testing drugs on the sick as haphazard and unreliable, particularly since the results being sought were often only symptomatic relief rather than eradication of the disease in its entirety.

Images of the Medicines

The concept of constitutional types has had a primary influence in prescribing. Since homeopathy views both patients and the medicines as psychosomatic images, it is capable of effecting symptoms which are part of the larger picture, symptoms the patient may have not reported or forgotten. The concept of constitution is a structural form determined by genetics, a fundamental predisposition or body type that remains consistent throughout life. It is suggested that a constitutional prescription does not change through life. So a fundamental constitutional prescription could be the same in both chronic and acute diseases and may be central throughout the course of a life's treatment.

It can become confusing if the homeopathic practitioner mistakes constitution with other aspects of treatment. While the constitutional remedy does not change, other influences which Hahnemann called miasmatic influences, may require other prescriptions. Miasms may be the residual influences from acquired infections, illnesses, or psychological traumas in the history.

Hahnemann also described one-sided cases in which the complexity of symptoms required prescribing for only the symptoms which were evident at the time. He felt these cases were rare. In practice, these are cases with extreme chemical and environmental sensitivities or chronic fatigue.

In modern times, homeopaths may speak of treating successive "layers." This theory was widely misused in recent homeopathic educational programs and became a poor excuse for not having given a correct prescription. In some ways it could be accused of enacting a similar form of symptomatic prescribing that homeopaths criticize other methods of. The problem results when the practitioner remains stuck in a rut, changing the remedy while claiming the constitution has changed, and not seeking consultation on the case when there is not an adequate response to treatment.

There is also the question of palliation, or the temporary alleviation of symptoms. While this is frowned upon by practicing homeopaths, it is an absolutely important part of health care, and homeopathy has a great deal to offer a patient who is suffering even when a cure is not possible.

These arguments concerning the focus of treatment are important. The outcome of a prescription can be based on how a practitioner directs his analysis. Some of the greatest homeopaths did not base the majority of their prescriptions on constitution, not even Hahnemann. Many successful prescriptions are based on peculiar characteristics of the case leading to a unique remedy.

The essence of homeopathic diagnosis from its vitalistic perspective is to understand the inner state of the patient and prescribe at the deepest level possible.

Dr. Eduard Von Grauvogl (1811–1877) introduced the concepts of constitution into homeopathy. Like the Salt, Sulphur, and Mercury of Paracelsus, he introduced a triune model for types. His constitutions were the Hydrogenoid, Oxygenoid, and Carbo-Nitrogenoid types. He followed Hahnemann in basing prescriptions on concomitant symptoms, those which are affected by general influences, such as weather or food cravings, that make the patient better or worse overall. A Hydrogenoid person is aggravated by the presence of water, whether baths or damp climates. Even the eating of foods such as fish or other water-dwellers can aggravate their condition. The Oxygenoid person is excessively thin despite adequate nutrition. They are sensitive to electrical fields, temperature changes, and fog. Von Grauvogl associated this constitution with syphilis, among other diseases. The Carbo-Nitrogenoid suffers from an inadequate absorption of oxygen. They may suffer from respiratory distress or asthma. They tend to be melancholic or even suicidal.

The reason constitution may not be well understood in American homeopathy is that Von Gravogl's *Textbook of Homeopathy,* which was published in English in 1870, was an extremely rare book until recently because the only edition was largely consumed by the Great Fire of Chicago. It is estimated that only four hundred copies survived.

Constitution can be mistaken for temperament. The temperament, however, represents our attitude, our perceptions of events, rather than a physical type. It is influenced by internal and external events. Its mutability contains our potentiality and degeneracy. The chronic effects of our responses to events in our lives represent an evolving process. Prescribing for the temperamental characteristics that distinguish us from others who share our constitutional state, even an identical twin, requires an individualized approach. Temperament is a major aspect of treatment in which we expect psychological change and maturity to develop. Prescribing based on temperament has broadened our experience of the many medicines that are used in treatment. The result in treatment may be the resolution of even serious physical pathology when the psychological temperament is the focus of the prescription.

A basic premise of homeopathic prescribing is matching the character of the patient with the character of the medicine. For this purpose "personality types" and descriptions are applied both to the patient and the substances used to treat them. The practitioner's task is to accurately assess the character of the patient and find a remedy with similar essential properties.

So a medicine, such as Sulphur for example, might be described as if it were the patient presenting in the clinic. Patients may be described as a "Sulphur type" because they represent the archetypal Sulphur symptomology commonly found.

The Sulphur patient can present as the ragged philosopher, who remains so entrenched in his ideas that he ignores his physical care and surroundings. He might keep seemingly messy piles of books and papers on his table, yet at a moment's notice, he can pull out the one paper that will support the theory he is dissertating on. Sulphur patients tend to be self-centered and rather arrogant, thinking they can resolve the secrets of humanity through complex study and research.

Or a Sulphur patient may present as more coarse and less subtle. They may be a worker who enjoys fiddling with mechanical tools—someone who is practical and enjoys using their hands.

Both types represent different clinical presentations of Sulphur. We don't want to become fixed on a singular description of a remedy however. It may be a characteristic symptom, something strange, rare, or peculiar that leads us to prescribe Sulphur or any other medicine. These are, in fact. the most important symptoms on which to prescribe. Generalizing about a patient can be misleading. By describing constitutional images or types, homeopathy is not attempting to simplify patients into categories. In fact, these descriptions of medicines are extremely complex, evolving as they express themselves in different stages of life and in diverse expressions of disease.

The commonality of the different Sulphur types may present through the physical characteristics. Sulphur types tend to produce skin lesions. They can have almost any skin disease. They are warm in general—in fact, they might stick their feet out of the bed covers at night. They may produce foul smelling discharges, often discolored yellow like the element Sulphur itself.

Sulphur is one of the most important medicines used in homeopathy, and its symptomology is vast. However, it is this ability to understand the underlying theme in Sulphur's image that leads the homeopath to consider its use. Then comes the tedious task of differentiating Sulphur from other remedies that share common symptoms.

Another common remedy type is *Pulsatilla nigrans,* the windflower. The person requiring Pulsatilla is also characterized as a warm patient, but Pulsatilla's personality is sensual and emotional. The two types both have yellow discharges, but where Sulphur's discharges are foul, burning and yellow, Pulsatilla's are thick, bland, and yellow. The Pulsatilla patient will weep easily, they are often sick from grief as they tend to yield in relationships and can become pathologically attached to their partners. Their moods are changeable. Pulsatilla is one of the main remedies for hormonal changes, particularly in premenstrual tension.

Calcarea carbonica, which comes from the oyster shell, is another common medicine. The people who need Calcarea share Sulphur's problem with their feet getting too warm at night and

Pulsatilla nigrans

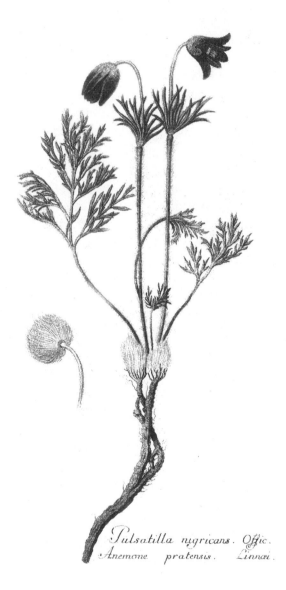

Pulsatilla nigricans. Offic.
Anemone pratensis. Linnæi.

[5 1]

having to stick them out of the covers. However Calcarea types are generally chilly; an earthy sort, they are methodical and plodding. These are the mainstays of any office, whose consistency and dependability are necessary to getting the job done. Where Sulphur would have one project after another half-baked, Calcarea is organized and efficient. *Calcarea carbonica* is remembered by the triad of symptoms: obesity, difficulty breathing on exertion, and constipation. The Calcarea type tends to be heavy-set and constipated; they huff and puff up steps and have to catch their breath at the landing.

It is also one of the most common medicines in chronic ear infections of children. As children they are little bruisers, solid, stocky children whose heads sweat at night. These children have particular fears, especially of ghosts, nightmares, and questions that seem prematurely serious for their age. They want to know where we came from and who God is. Other children do not question their existence at such a young age.

Since specific mental or emotional symptoms are primary in analyzing a case for a homeopathic prescription, one can differentiate based on a symptom such as jealousy, grief, anger, or a specific phobia or delusion. One of the most effective medicines in suicidal depression is *Aurum metallicum* (Gold). Aurum patients have a long history of being extremely serious. They take their work seriously and feel a great responsibility for their actions. So if they fail at anything it is devastating. They become extremely anxious and irritable and will have moments when they see a way out. They may come to a ledge and think, this may be my chance! Or while driving they may become so involved in their anguish that they drive faster until they lose control at a curve.

In the past, gold was associated with the sun and with the heart. Aurum is a major homeopathic remedy in the treatment of heart disease. In Orthodox medicine, Gold injections are used in the treatment of arthritis. In homeopathy, gold has been found useful in arthritis, as well as having successfully treated bone tumors. One can see by these diverse effects that to simply inject arthritic nodes with Gold salts would fail to understand the true relationship of Gold to arthritis. For patients who require Aurum, the sun has gone from their life. If we understand the essential character and effects of the medicine, *Aurum metallicum,* we can administer it in a way that acts more profoundly.

Specific delusions of the mind are recorded as having been cured through homeopathic treatment. As a modern psychological development in homeopathy, these observations of delusions have been incorporated into a more comprehensive understanding of delusional and repetitive outlooks on life. Misunderstandings and misperceptions, as well as psychotic states, may be considered as delusions. So someone who complains that they have always been cheated and that everyone is against them may need one of the medicines referenced under "Delusions persecuted."

To understand each reference listed under delusions, we must understand the context of the delusion in the psychology of the remedy as a whole. It is the pathological, limiting expression of the delusion which is to be studied, not its positive context. Remedies associated with joyfulness are listed not because joy is a disease but because someone who only expresses joy exclusively or excessively is perhaps denying their suffering. In Chinese medicine there is a saying, "excessive joy damages the heart."

Dogmatism may be found under "Religious affections" or "Dictatorial." A person who believes they see the demons or the devil may benefit from Belladonna, *Pulsatilla nigrans,* or the metals Zinc or Platinum.

Platinum has been used both in patients with violent impulses to kill and also in nymphomania. It is seen more commonly in persons who are haughty, proud, and secretive, as if they valued themselves, as the most valuable person on earth, just as Platinum is the most valuable of metals.

The chronic mental state of Belladonna pathology includes violent impulses, as well as its more acute symptoms of common fevers, convulsions, and delerium. In fact, Hahnemann's insights into Belladonna's use as a preventative and treatment for scarlet fever in the 1800s led to the widespread use of homeopathy in that disease, with much greater success than orthodox methods.

Zinc is used in neurological disorders, often involving the central nervous system. It is one of the most common remedies in restless leg syndrome.

A wide range of fears are listed in homeopathic literature; claustrophobia, fear of the dark, of death, of disease, and of going insane are just a few.

The preponderance of vast numbers of symptoms in the homeopathic *Materia Medica* describe an entire range of human experience, from the common neurotic to the deepest recesses of human suffering.

Healing the Emotions

Since healthy relationships are essential to the well-being of people, we find a great difficulty arising from the inability to express love. Grief and dissatisfaction arising from misunderstandings in relationships are at often the core of illness. So many problems can be antedated to a period in which there was a separation or loss. Abuse and abandonment are critical wounds that may affect development for years to come. Yet each of us responds to trauma in a unique way. Two children of the same parents will react to similar stresses each according to his or her unique nature.

Sexuality plays a key role in the genesis of relationships as an adult. Often in a homeopathic interview, the expressions relating to sexuality are keys to understanding the instinctual motivations of the overall personality. Suppression of sexual desire, as well as sexual dysfunction and mental disorders surrounding sexual activity, are addressed.

We mentioned Platinum as being used in both psychotic impulses and nymphomania. One patient seen for ovarian tumors admitted to having secret impulses to kill her children, which she could not explain. On further questioning about her sexuality, she became angered and insisted she was just like anyone else. She lived in an extremely conservative Christian community. Her husband was a member of the John Birch Society. It seemed she did not necessarily agree with him but that it was something she endured.

What I heard from her becoming defensive was that the strength of her unexpressed sexual life, whatever it may have been, was driving her a little mad. Since Platinum is known to treat ovarian tumors, and is one of the few remedies listed under both impulses to kill and complaints from the suppression of sexual desire, I presumed her anger at the questions on her sexuality was due to her inability to express it in the conservative society in which she lived. It is not so much a comment about her community but the way in which she unconsciously compensated within those expectations.

A dose of Platinum acted beautifully. She did not return for a year, and that was to accompany a relative. She reported that all her ovarian complaints had resolved and she no longer felt anger toward her children. This is what we would want in a curative response.

This shows how medicines can affect our lives. To most it is almost incomprehensible that medicines can actually act to heal or cure when we have been so indoctrinated into expecting medicines to control symptoms.

Homeopathy can be utilized to great advantage in conjunction with counseling in these cases. Homeopathy works as a feedback mechanism, mirroring the unconscious impulses, while counseling helps to integrate the unfoldment of the emotions and place it constructively in context. Learning the tools of communication is essential for healthy relationships. This should be a priority in primary and secondary education. We are taught about DNA in school before we know about human anatomy and physiology. We are taught too little about skills necessary to function as an adult.

Communication, economics, health, and disease are essential foundations of knowledge that are often superseded by the educational orientation to job skills. If basic health and psychological skills were taught before adult relationships were established, many mistakes and subsequent illnesses could be avoided.

[55]

Homeopathic medicine is a therapeutic tool that addresses the nature of disease and the interpenetration of mind/body relationship at a profound level. In the context of treatment, the many influences, both environmental and endogenous, are important. The goal is to understand the human system in such a way that we can aid in the processes of healing rather than disrupting them. Homeopathy offers perhaps the most diverse model in Western medicine for addressing these concerns, and it is one that has been confirmed clinically, sustaining itself throughout the world as a small voice amidst the big guns of medicine.

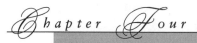

Barberry and the Treatment of Sexual Trauma

*We must describe the other half of man in order that
the physician may understand him as a whole. Although
this aspect is invisible, it may be seen in the light of nature.
It is the same when we hear a bell on a dark night.
We cannot see it, and yet we see the work of the bell;
that is, we hear it, for every work has a light in which it
can be seen. Do not be downcast that all things are not
clear as day, but consider how secretive God is. And when
we learn something, we discover that we erroneously call
the invisible things invisible, for all works teach us that
they have a cause. We see the work visibly before our eyes,
and once we have investigated its author, that is also
visible to us.*

—Paracelsus

In each person is a secret, sometimes long forgotten, that they hide even to themselves. Likewise, in every medicine are healing properties, which correspond to our ills yet are often disregarded. To call attention to what is unseen and reveal its nature is the basis of the Law of Similars. It is a matter of respecting the subtle properties of life, the wisdom of the infinitesimal, those processes that are beyond the scope of our senses. There is no way to fully know the patient or the medicines; we are led by clues and associations. We make inferences and determine from past experience our conclusions and best judgment.

When we study a person or their corresponding medicine, it as if we are looking at a jewel through different facets, trying to see its inner workings from the outside. Most of the facets are invisible to us, or are clouded over. Because we try to find one facet that is visible to our perception, that fits our limited knowledge, each of us inevitably has a different interpretation of the situation. It's difficult to come from the inside, to understand the healing function. The light of nature is a natural phenomenon. It is everywhere.

It is similar to the way we might try to understand a close friend. There are so many people walking down the street, yet we recognize our friend by their walk or that funny hat they wear that we never really liked, or by any of those things that make up an individual.

It is the same with our petty judgments and gossip. Our opinions are based on one-sided interpretations. We see only the results of others' behavior, and hear only innuendoes of misperceived actions. If we are to have compassion for others, we must look at the underlying history of others' actions. Perhaps the reason for that individual being such a creep is that some of the most important people in their lives treated them the same way. Maybe they were beaten down, made to feel like no one could ever love them, or that they were to blame for something horrible that happened to them. It becomes a self-fulfilling prophecy. Those who have been abused look for some way to escape from the blame they inflict upon themselves. They wonder, if only they had done something differently, then maybe it wouldn't have happened.

The Unstated Origins
of Disease

We need to see behind the mask. It demands being aware of how to communicate in a way that doesn't threaten others. Behind our defenses is the repressed desire for love and appreciation. Our anger is often misdirected towards the innocent, hiding the fears and hurts. Our sadness is unexpressed, tears well up at a sad movie when the soundtrack triggers our emotions, but we are often incapable of responding honestly in human encounters.

This sociopathology we see around us arises from the chain of inhumanity that repeats itself from the imprints of past generations. When Sigmund Freud introduced his trauma theory, it was so unacceptable to the medical society of his times that he was forced to couch it in symbolic rather than direct terms, such as the Oedipal complex. If we were only aware of the extent of abuse and trauma, we would be in constant pain at the shocking pervasiveness of evil that exists in our society. In recent years, more and more information has been accumulating about the depth and breadth of this problem. Sexual abuse is being reported and studied with increasing frequency. Recent studies suggest that as many as one in three women and one in five men have been sexually abused. This sickness in our society is not being adequately addressed, either by the legal system itself or by our communities.

Many sexual abuse situations are cases of incest. What is the definition of incest? Incest can be defined as any sexual abuse of a child by a relative or other person in a position of trust and authority over the child. It is the violation of the child where he or she "lives," literally or metaphorically. A child molested by a stranger can run home for help and comfort. A victim of incest cannot.

Incest and other abuse victims also suffer from Posttraumatic Stress Disorder. This is the same disorder that has been identified in war veterans and victims of torture. The symptoms include, but are not limited to, amnesia, nightmares, and flashbacks. People who have Posttraumatic Stress Disorder may "leave their bodies" during the abuse, and they may dissociate for decades, long after the abuse ends. Most sexual abuse victims have sexual problems as adults and many have eating disorders. There is a distinct inability to nourish or be nourished.

Perhaps the greatest tragedy is that most of the people who have suffered abuse have been threatened in their lives and told to not say anything. So the suffering lies hidden in secrets.

SECRETS OF BERBERIS VULGARIS: THE HOLY THORN

Berberis vulgaris, or barberry, is a bushy shrub that grows to a height of three to eight feet. The stem woods, pith, bark, and flowers are yellow. Berberis is the Arabic name of the fruit, signifying a shell because the leaves are glossy like the inside of an oyster shell. The Italians call it the "holy thorn" because it is thought to have formed part of the crown of thorns made for Christ.

Cows, sheep, and goats eat the shrub; horses and swine refuse it, and birds seldom touch the fruit because of its acidity.

Gerard, in *The Herbal or General History of Plants,* speaks of Berberis as being useful against hot burnings and choleric fevers, allaying the heat of the blood and liver. He mentions the fruits and berries as an antidote for hot flashes, the "bloody flux," or dysentery, and any superfluous bleeding.

Dr. Hesse, one of the early German homeopaths, proved *Berberis vulgaris,* and published his findings in the *Journal for Materia Medica* in 1834. The first translations appeared in *Jahr's Manual,* which was published in English in 1834. James Tyler Kent, M.D., one of the most influential homeopathic physicians, developed psychological descriptions for clinical applications of medicines at the turn of the century. He states that few of the mental states of Berberis are known. For the most part, the use of Berberis has been limited to acute prescribing for kidney infections and gallstone colic.

It was through clinical experience that I was able to discover the range of action of this wonderful medicine.

A forty-seven-year-old woman came to my office complaining of sinus problems that had begun after she found out her brother had an incurable disease. He subsequently died of primary pulmonary hypertension at age thirty-seven. At first she only spoke of her presenting symptoms, but soon, as I let her know that her history was important to me, she described her experiences of multiple personality, which she'd had since childhood. Her disorder was misdiagnosed until later life. At age thirty she was diagnosed as manic-depressive, and put on lithium. Her other brother also had a diagnosis of multiple personality disorder and was an alcoholic. She was a recovering marijuana "addict." She had quit coffee, which she felt suppressed her feelings. Finally, she revealed a critical piece of her story, that she had been beaten at sixteen months and she suspected that her father sexually molested her. During her teens he was sexually aggressive toward her.

She had been fearful since her brother's death a year earlier and had been unable to do her work. She felt a combination of anxiety and insecurity. She felt scared in grocery stores. She said she was pessimistic and cranky. She didn't get angry easily because she was afraid she'd get really angry if she did. "Poor me," she said to herself. She always kept secrets from people. In fact, during our conversation she stopped and asked if it was okay to talk about this, because the psychiatrist who had originally diagnosed her had told her it was better not to mention it to anyone because they wouldn't understand. She told me it was the first time she had shared her story since then.

She had four separate personalities. Susan was youngest and maintained the knowledge of early traumas. Diana appeared only when things were going well. Sharon was the original personality who didn't know of the others. Terra was the original split from Diana.

A month earlier she suddenly felt extremely cold. She had a sinus infection that had been chronic for two years. It was diagnosed as a staphylococcal infection. She had a creamy yellow nasal discharge, but no head pain. A bronchial cough remained since she quit smoking. She had chronic kidney and bladder infections with an urging to urinate and heavy burning before urination. Yet her urine tests were negative.

Chronic recurrent urinary symptoms are a red flag. Often symptoms can be a natural defense in areas where we feel we have been violated. There were pains in her abdomen (presumably from the bladder) and in her back behind the kidneys. Her menses were normal. She had low blood pressure and body temperature. She craved sweets, oranges, and bananas; as a child she ate ice. She was plagued by chronic constipation.

Her food cravings told me more about her metabolism. She slept on her stomach, never on her back, showing how she protected herself at night. Her dreams might have told more, or may have led us on a goose chase through the discharges of the unconscious, but during our conversation I mostly listened. Perhaps no one else really listened to her. I asked questions only to allow her to clarify and release as much as possible, to let her know that what she had to tell was important, that I cared about her and what she said.

She was the single parent of a seven-year-old daughter. She said her "hysteric body" reacted to emotions, yet she didn't remember having sex. Her sexual experiences remain coalesced in the memory of a separate personality.

I chose *Berberis vulgaris* as an initial prescription in this case because it is one of the main remedies for chronic kidney and bladder infections and the associated pains. It is also listed as a minor remedy under sinus infections. Interestingly, Dr. Marjorie Blackie, Queen Elizabeth's former family physician, mentions it as being useful in "contradictory, changeable personalities."

The case had many elements of what Hahnemann described as the Sycotic miasm. The miasms are a theory of chronic disease in homeopathy in which the chronic effects of a suppressed or incompletely treated disease are related to subsequent syndromes. For example, the sequela of gonorrhea might include the common symptoms of Reiter's syndrome; urinary inflammation (urethritis), eye inflammation (conjunctivitis), and arthritis.

Some of the patterns associated with the sequela of gonorrhea may also include sinus infections, allergies, and a psychological state of secretiveness. I certainly considered giving her Medorrhinum, which is a specific remedy for the sycotic or gonorrheal miasm. She did have the classic cravings for oranges and a history of eating ice, which corresponded to the symptomology of Medorrhinum. She even slept on her abdomen, which is also a characteristic symptom to indicate Medorrhinum. But I may have led the interview too much, asking for symptoms confirming a well-known medicine. I felt if she required Medorrhinum, she would express more excessive sexuality rather than inhibition.

I also thought of *Thuja occidentalis,* the arbor vitae tree, for this case. Thuja has many of the characteristics of Medorhinum. Its profile incorporates the psychological state of secretiveness and it is one of the main medicines in the treatment of the abused. The secretiveness of Thuja originates more from a feeling of insecurity and worthlessness. The patients feel the need to fit in and hide their pasts. In Thuja patients, you get the feeling that there isn't much to this person; they seem too ordinary, complacent and depressed. Medorrhinum is the opposite. The secretiveness is more an expression of a truer darkness, of people whose behavior challenges morality and who relish their ability to shock and offend others' conservativeness.

However, I was not satisfied with Thuja or any other commonly prescribed medicine. I have since come to the conclusion that Berberis is very close to Thuja in its symptomology.

I finally gave Berberis because of its exact correspondence to the physical symptomology and some insights into its psychological states that I will discuss later. After all, in homeopathy it doesn't quite work to look up multiple personalities and come up with some simple solution. It takes some digging to understand why and what put this person in this state.

The two week follow-up took me by surprise. The physical aspects of her case had largely resolved, in particular the bladder and kidney pain, as well as the sinusitis. However, the most remarkable aspect of her response was a noticeable integration of several of the personalities, and a subsequent reemergence of the personality that represented her original split, Terra. Terra was the aspect of herself that she described as whole, the predecessor of her lost self.

Six weeks after her initial visit the integration of her personality continued to progress. By this visit, she had only conscious dialogues with Terra rather than missing periods of time in which she was unconsciously dominated. She continued to do well, without any repetition of the remedy. I then referred her to a psychologist who specialized in the field of multiple personalities.

In another case, a thirty-eight-year-old woman visited me complaining of internal hemorrhoids with excessive bleeding. She had pain in the rectum, which was made worse when she was sitting. Four months earlier she emitted a cup of blood with her stool for a couple of days. This recurred at Thanksgiving, which she associated with eating meat.

Twelve years ago she had kidney and bladder infections and was coughing up blood, though I never found out why.

She was a lovely woman and her voice was so quiet, I almost had to strain to understand her. She said she suffered from depression. Her family was abusive when she was growing up. Her mother had been hospitalized for a nervous breakdown. She stated she was raised as an only child after age five when her brother joined the navy. She had asthma between ages five and twelve. She gained weight until age twelve. Her father was an alcoholic and violent. He left when she was twelve.

She was raped repeatedly between the ages of seven and ten by a family "friend."

She was withdrawn and had been a recluse for the past year. She tended to hold in her anger and she felt bitter. She felt heat rising to her head and she felt as if she was going to have a stroke. She cried a lot, although she didn't even cry during her labor. She felt apathetic.

Ten days earlier she began coughing up blood after being exposed to the cold. She felt cold in general. She felt heat in her left breast and liver. Her menses were irregular.

She had been sexually active since age eighteen. She was unable to have an orgasm until she left her first husband and then had six affairs after her marriage ended. At that time she had a ravenous appetite for sex and was attracted to abusive men. In the past several years she had no sexual desire. She feared that her daughter would die and she would be left alone. Her hands trembled visibly. She had anxiety attacks and heart palpitations. I gave her *Mercurius corrosivus*.

Mercurius, which was indicated for her bleeding hemorrhoids, is also known in homeopathy as a medicine for extremely closed individuals who hold the mysteries of their lives inside.

Twelve days later she returned. She was sleeping through the night and her palpitations had ended. The coughing had stopped. Her bowel movements were normal. The stool was normal without any pain. The heat in her liver was not as intense and the heat in her breast was almost gone. Her rectum still hurt when she sat but not as badly. The night sweats were gone. She felt her mental state was unchanged. I felt this was a good response so far, so I allowed the medicine to continue its action.

Three days later she returned with pain below her sternum, which was reduced by lying on her back. Her eyes had begun oozing yellow mucous two days earlier and were bloodshot. There was no longer blood in her stool. She got occasional nausea, but wasn't regurgitating. She was chilly and her skin was jaundiced.

I had to differentiate the cause of the jaundice. In this case, because of localized pain upon palpation of the gallbladder, I determined that the colic pain and jaundice occurred from a bile duct obstruction.

The question for me here was, what was the effect of the Mercurius? There were no changes in the mental state, so the prescription may have had an acute effect without affecting the chronic state. Or perhaps it was acting superficially, suppressing the underlying chronic condition temporarily and leading to a crisis. Or was this some sort of healing crisis? Was the liver obstruction an attempt by the body to eliminate toxins that were overwhelming its capacity?

These are the questions we must ask ourselves at every follow-up, even when a crisis isn't occurring. What is the effect of the prescription, not only regarding the chief complaint, but also to the whole life of the person? How does the effect of the

[65]

medicine upon its intended target of symptoms relate to its effect on the myriad of unexpressed symptoms?

In this situation, I prescribed Berberis in the botanical tincture. This may seem confusing to some. Homeopaths tend to pride themselves on the use of potentized substances rather than crude extractions. For me, homeopathy isn't just about the potentization of medicines, it is about understanding how to prescribe. Any substance, whether pharmaceutical, botanical, or from any source can be applied by the Law of Contraries to control physiology, or by the Law of Similars to catalyze healing.

The question of dosage concerns both the subtle properties of matter and also the toxicological side effects of improper use of crude substances. All matter has its subtle effects. A homeopathic dose or a botanical tincture can carry its effects. But the purpose of homeopathic and alchemical preparations of substances has been to remove the dross of a substance's gross action and accentuate its effects on more subtle and powerful systemic action.

So in giving the tincture, I may have focused the prescription at a physiological situation, but because I was prescribing homeopathically I understood that deeper effects of Berberis might take effect.

Soon after taking the Berberis tincture, the patient's jaundice and pain subsided. Within the next month, her friends noticed an entire change had occurred in her life. She was able to overcome her depression and withdrawal and had made plans to start a new business. Her way of seeing her world had shifted. This is what we seek in treatment. This change in life tells us we have been able to reach a deeper level of healing. We have affected the root.

Berberis vulgaris is a medicine for the secret wound inside. We all contain separate personalities within us. In cases where there has been severe physical or sexual abuse, as is the case in all multiple personality disorder patients, the split becomes too great and normal conscious activities can coalesce under the direction of unconscious aspects of the subpersonalities.

The first case led me to examine the cases where I had prescribed Berberis previously, particularly in the cases of chronic

Berberis vulgaris

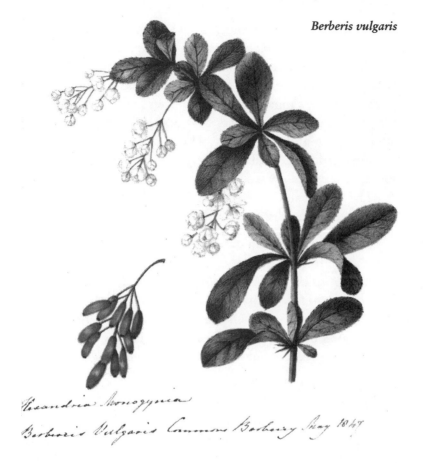

Pecandria Monogynia

Berberis Vulgaris Common Barberry May 1847

vaginitis and urinary tract infections. As I discovered that many
of these cases had histories of sexual abuse, I came to the conclusion that these physical symptoms may be acting as a defense
mechanism for the emotional wounds of the patient. I hypoth-
esized that Berberis may indeed treat the deeper wounds, of
which the physical aspects were only a manifestation. Since my
initial presentation of these ideas at a conference in 1992, they
have been consistently confirmed.

The essence of the wound that requires Berberis is a secret
that remains hidden even to the patients themselves. The medicine combines the symptomology of urogenital inflammation,
suppression of emotions, and secretiveness. It lies somewhere

[67]

between the symptomologies of two other medicines, Staphysagria and *Thuja occidentalis*. In Staphysagria, the anger lies close to the surface manifesting as trembling and quivering of the voice. In Berberis, the origins are often no longer accessible to the conscious mind. They lie quiescent, coalesced in a conflict that creates fatigue, withdrawal, and psychosomatic expressions of pain and discomfort. The pain itself is not clear. It wanders, radiating in different directions from the kidney, liver, joints, and sexual organs.

The mental state is described in the first homeopathic text translated into English, *Jahr's Manual,* published in 1848,

> Mental languor, with difficulty to collect one's thoughts ... Indifferent, sad mood. Calm, sometimes even apathetic. Striking melancholy, and irresistible want of disposition to talk, with silent longing of a spiritual nature. Disposition to weep. One feels vexed and even tired of life. Anxious mood, with great fearfulness and tendency to start. Great anguish and uneasiness.

It is listed in the *Materia Medica* under Agony, desire for death; Instability of ideas; Indifference and Insanity.

Barthel, a modern author, lists Berberis under Ailments from suppressed sexual desire; Enjoyment absent (during sexual activity); Aversion to coition; Orgasm delayed; Generally worse during and after coition; and Premature aging.

Constantine Hering, the father of American homeopathy, wrote of Berberis:

> [It has] suppressed desire with long delayed thrill, and frequent cutting and stitching in parts during coition. Complete want of pleasurable sensations during coition. Coition is painful. Indicated in Ovarian disease.

E.A. Farrington mentions in his *Clinical Materia Medica* of 1887, Berberis's usefulness in inflammation of the peritoneum that lines the cavity of the abdomen, also known as peritonitis and metritis, which is inflammation of the uterus lining. It is interesting to observe how early the homeopathic physicians were far ahead of their time in being able to objectively deal with sexuality and understand its importance in human health and function. Though they held that ethical behavior was an important aspect of a healthy inner state, their ability to describe the consequences of sexual diseases was coupled with a realistic observation of human sexual experience.

The physical characteristics of *Berberis vulgaris* are well documented. A modern author and good friend, Matthew Wood, notes:

> (The pulse is described) in some patients as "full, hard, and rapid." These are usually the more recent cases where there are symptoms of fullness and heat: swollen, hot, red tissues. In the more chronic patients the pulse is more likely to be low, wiry and rapid; the face is pallid, with sunken eyes surrounded by blue or blackish circles, puffy underneath. In most of the cases I have seen, the tongue was red, especially along the edges, sometimes with yellow coating in the middle, and often with red protuberances.

Besides the chronic urinary tract and liver disorders, Berberis is known for treating hemorrhoids and anal fistulas, rheumatic problems with wandering pains, and general fatigue or adrenal exhaustion.

Berberis vulgaris is in the same botanical family as Goldenseal *(Hydrastis canadensis)* and Oregon Grape (*Berberis aquifolium* or Mahonia). They all contain high concentrations of Berberine, which is a botanical active ingredient used for its antibiotic properties. While such mechanical properties of Berberis are a virtue, we see through developing our understanding of the individual plant nature that we can develop a deeper understanding of the true healing properties of our medicines.

[69]

Chapter Five

THE DISEASE OF SEPARATION

Healing
I am ill because of wounds to the soul,
to the deep emotional self
and the wounds to the soul take a long, long time,
only time can help
and patience, and a certain difficult repentance
long, difficult repentance, realization of life's mistake,
and the freeing oneself
from the endless repetition of the mistake
which mankind at large has chosen to sanctify.

—D.H. Lawrence

[71]

Our nomadic ancestors return in us. The cowboys of the nineteenth century now roam the range in diesel trucks. Americans change their residences every four years. The single mother, divorce, and abortion rates soar. Adolescents are treated as children. Their early knowledge of adulthood is accompanied by a lack of wisdom from guidance. Girls approach their menstrual periods at earlier ages. Our gestation period is the longest of any known species. Our sense of adulthood and independence from the family takes ever longer as requirements for adequate education to compete in the marketplace steadily increase. As our gestation in adolescence is prolonged, so is our rebellion and inability to form coherent ties with our pasts. The rites of passage have been misplaced so that they are enacted within the group from a sense of nihilism rather than purpose.

For the first time in our evolution, physicians whom women entrusted their care to would advise them not to breastfeed, not to hold their children when they were crying. Hospitals separate mothers from their children at birth. This is possibly the most misanthropic act in the history of medicine, and with long-term effects on mass populations. Our generations became the most significantly unbonded in the history of mankind, based on medical advice. This inability to bond is passed from generation to generation. The inability to bond has effects which present themselves not only in our relationships, but in substance abuse, criminality, and the inability to function with honesty.

We create our homes, our architecture, our societies, and our values that focus and direct our lives. It is our instincts that form the base of emotional reactions and sense of security. The animal instinct responds from the amygdala and basal ganglia of our brain forming our response to the environment. Do we feel comfortable that we can rest in our milieu?

We became the industrial nations where mountains were crushed to make the roads and parking lots. Our reflections were seen in steel and glass, instead of water. We bonded to whatever was shown from an electrical box that told us our visions. Our primary disease is separation, the lack of being rooted, of not feeling at home, in the world, in our bodies, and in ourselves. It is a homesickness. In primitive medicine, this was called a loss of soul. The shaman's task was to travel in the spirit world to find the lost self, to bring it back, and merge it with our lives. It is the attempt to find meaning.

In Leviticus, it is mentioned that the lepers were cast out of society. That same sense has pervaded our alienation from the group as ennui and apathy. In the year 1226, in France alone, there were 2,000 houses for the care of lepers. Leprosy persisted in the West until the advent of regular bathing and cotton clothing in the fifteenth century. The disease most frequently appeared as elephantiasis, though it was undoubtedly misdiagnosed, often as other diseases such as psoriasis or syphilis. The disease of the skin emerged again in the Middle Ages as St. Anthony's Fire or malignant erysipelas. St. Anthony, the protector of those afflicted with this disease, is represented with a fire beside him.

The skin represents our most superficial relationship to the environment. Like the lungs, kidneys and bowels it functions to eliminate toxins. Skin is central to our appearance and its lesions are great concern for self-respect. How natural it is that teenagers develop acne as their hormones change, as a means to ward off too close an emotional interaction. It is as if the body is producing a barrier until emotional development can catch up with the maturation process.

Yet again, we try to eliminate all signs of disease. Skin lesions are treated as symptoms rather than expressions of an internal disease. Medical history is a record of attempts to inhibit this expression. So eventually our defense mechanisms are perverted. What was a superficial inflammation emerges as internal proliferation, the malfunction of eliminatory passageways, cystic and tumor formations. These were the basis for Hahnemann's idea of psora, the primary miasm. The word psora came from the story of leprosy in Leviticus, which for Hahnemann represented the primordial example of a unifying principle which underlied the diseases of mankind.

It is the multifaceted expression of this inflammation and its elimination that plagues us with the secondary manifestations of functional disease. It presents as diseases that are undefined.

Allergies are our reaction to the world around us. Allergic reactions, inflammation, and autoimmune diseases are all over-reactions to what should be normal.

Allergies represent our inability to find our place in our world. We treat them without understanding their message, without solving their meaning. So they return again and again throughout our lives, as environmental illnesses, anxieties, or eruptions. All symptoms seek resolution and harmony. We seek some quiet sense of belonging.

This is the multi-headed monster. Our sense of not belonging to the group expresses the archetypes of the scapegoat and the outcast. We see the world as something that happens to us, rather than an act we participate in. Our point of view becomes a defense to what threatens us, instead of one of many possible responses, a fixed reaction. Then we reinforce the expectations of others. We become crystallized. The element of surprise is missing.

The problem is consatellated in our myths of the outlaw, the loner, and the crucifixion. It is the story of Hansel and Gretel, when they awake to find the birds have eaten all the crumbs. Whether from social situations or economic influences, we may find ourselves in unfamiliar territory, a misplaced geography, lost in the wilderness. The flora opposes our imprinted sense of comfort. Even on a sunny day our prospects become dark and threatening.

In a society that is so displaced, where the bonding between parents and children is disrupted, we find the need for *Carbo animalis*. It is for the pathology generated from the loss of home and instinct.

Carbo Animalis

I have found this remedy to be prominent in addressing the disease of loneliness.

The clinical basis of *Carbo animalis* has historically been focused on its use in fulminant cancers, in which the lymph glands have been enlarged. It is a remedy described in cases of cancer of the uterus and breast. It is mentioned as suited to old persons, greatly debilitated, with blueness of the skin. It is indicated in the last stage of pneumonia, bronchitis, and tuberculosis. Weakness of nursing women is an indication.

Carbo animalis is prepared from a thick piece of ox-hide

placed between red-hot coals, where it must remain as long as it burns with a flame. Then it is quickly put between plates of stone to put a stop to the combustion. If it is allowed to cool gradually in the air, most of the carbon is consumed.

Carbon is the base of organic matter, the form of life on earth. Carbon creates organic life forms. It binds with hydrogen, oxygen, nitrogen, and itself to structure a whole range of organic compounds. Its versatility far exceeds that of the inorganic minerals. It is present in the air as carbon dioxide, which plants absorb to utilize the carbon in creating structure, liberating oxygen in exchange.

Carbo animalis is indicated not only in cancer but also in cases with a previous history of cancer.

What is the basis for cancer in generation after generation? How does cancer arise from the poisons in our environment? Cancer is a disease of unconsciousness. Like a virus, many of which can be the instigator of tumors, it is unrecognized by the body, until its development impedes the function of an organ or creates pain through displacement.

When Albert Schweitzer was asked if he had encountered cancer among his native patients in Africa, he replied that he had never seen a case until the white man arrived. Africans do not get skin cancer in any significant numbers, presumably because the pigmentation of their skin protects them from the carcinogenic effects of the sun. But then why do African Americans get skin cancer?

When we look in the homeopathic pharmacopoeia for medicines listed under homesickness, we find *Carbo animalis,* Bryonia, Capsicum (red pepper), Ignatia amara, Magnesium muriaticum, Mercury, and Phosphoric acid as the main medicines utilized in this psychological state.

Each medicine has its own uniquely associated mental states. As we develop the nature of each of these medicines from the homeopathic provings on healthy experimenters, we find the experience of homesickness. Then as we confirm those relationships in clinical practice, we begin to see patterns arising that express the common expressions of the state that requires that medicine.

The *Carbo animalis* patient becomes absorbed. They have anxiety when they close their eyes, anxiety in the dark, anxiety with debility, anxiety driving them from place to place.

They feel as if they are in a deserted town. They can have dreams of wandering. They experience indolence and aversion to work. Their jobs are burdens. It is a sense of ennui and tedium. They fear narrow places, vaults, churches, and cellars. They desire light.

These are the actual experiences. Then how do we see them? How do we recognize this medicine in our patients, our friends?

Much of the minor symptomology of *Carbo animalis* appears to me to represent the symptoms of functional diseases. These diseases are not readily diagnosable, frequently recurring, or changing in symptomology. They do not represent significant pathology.

Based on the psychological state, with confirming physical characteristics, I found *Carbo animalis* indicated in cases throughout the life history of those who have been displaced. They are driven not by a desire for change of place or travel, but rather their circumstances evolve out of loss of connection. Their anxiety and hurried states come from never feeling protected and nourished. *Carbo animalis* may be indicated in cases of abuse, divorce, and bereavement, as well as in military brats who have moved frequently and in the chemically addicted. In many situations where attachment and bonding have been disrupted, Carbo animalis may be indicated.

Separation can come at any age. For example, I saw a two-year-old boy who was adopted, and whose adoptive mother was recently divorced. They had recently moved to Colorado. The mother had no friends from her past and would not speak to her former husband except regarding practical matters concerning the care of their son. His life was a series of sudden detachments from those who were closest. Despite his friendly disposition I felt his life situation had influenced his health. His chronic colds and earaches resolved under *Carbo animalis*.

In another case, a fifty-two-year-old woman who was experiencing mood swings consulted me. She was on estrogen replacement therapy after a partial hysterectomy in 1972, due to a benign tumor. Five years previously, she had a mastectomy due to breast cancer. She had experienced stiffness for six months in her hands, knees, and hips. She was fatigued most of the time. She'd had short-term memory loss for the past five years.

She was divorced after ten years of marriage. She felt she could never depend on her former husband. In the course of their marriage, she moved fifteen times. She was impatient and angry, which was worse when she drove. Due to the history of cancer, frequent moving, and arthritic symptoms, I prescribed *Carbo animalis*. Her anger and fatigue were relieved within a few weeks and her arthritis began to be diminished. By the third visit, her joint pain was gone.

Soon I was able to see the common need for *Carbo animalis*. A sixty-two-year-old woman, who had moved to be with her daughter after her husband died, came to see me. She worked at a large computer software company where she found herself experiencing severe allergies. She complained of fatigue, that she was "just not herself." She had frequent colds and recurring bronchitis since moving. Her legs cramped. She felt better in the damp rain of the East and worse in the dry air of Colorado. She reminisced about how beautiful her life in the Bronx had been. Colorado and the Rocky Mountains just did not comfort her. She felt people around her were draining her energy. She wanted to be alone. She was always afraid her house in the East would burn down. She worried about things she could not control. She thought she would lose her mind or die of cancer.

After *Carbo animalis*, she felt energetic and exclaimed, "Maybe living in Colorado isn't so bad." She began walking and jogging. Her allergies were not affecting her. The cramps in her legs were almost all gone. She no longer felt homesick.

[77]

Another medicine we must consider in the feeling of being outcast is *Hura braziliensis*. Hura has been used in leprosy, where the skin feels as if it were tight and bound. The theme of the outcast and the leper is closely associated with this remedy. Hura is a member of the Euphorbiacae family that includes *Acalypha indica, Croton tiglium,* Euphorbium, Jatropa, Mancinella, and Stillingia. These are highly caustic plants that cause great skin and mucous membrane irritation.

Hura is listed in the literature under the following mental symptoms: Forsaken feeling; Delusions they are despised; Deserted; Feels alone in the world; Delusions they are repudiated by their relatives; Forsaken with a sense of isolation; Thinks of Death; and feeling unfortunate.

Hura is a medicine for the deepest of depressions in which hopelessness predominates the landscape of the mind. It can be compared with the indications for Gold *(Aurum metallicum)* with its deep sense of responsibility and doom, or Antimony *(Antimonium crudum),* which is indicated in a person with a great sense of failure. In these medicines, we would expect to see some generation of emotion. In Hura patients, there are often none.

A middle-aged woman who I had treated for many years had moved away to the western slope of Colorado, to a beautiful dark town in a canyon. She had three children and had hoped that by living near their father there would be a more cohesive support system for the family.

She soon found she had made a mistake. She experienced rejection from her former husband and subsequently from the community. She lived with this burden for seven years before returning to her former home.

She came to my office complaining of a staphylococcus infection on her face that was threatening to affect her eyes. The common name for this infection is impetigo. Some of the main remedies used in treating impetigo are Dulcamara, Black Walnut, Graphites, and *Rhus toxidendron.* But my experience told me that this was a chronic situation that would only be served by addressing its root.

She had returned to her former home out of a deep sense of despair, having felt she had lived in rejection by her community all these years. There were many times in which she was unable to function due to her sadness and subsequently she suffered several misfortunes including physical accidents and financial woes.

She responded beautifully to a dose of Hura, which lifted her spirits and resolved the long-term impetigo. Even though Hura is not listed under impetigo, it contains both the mental state and the characteristic description of skin eruptions that matched her condition. We may want to add Hura to our list of impetigo medicines. But more importantly, Hura helped her to move forward in her life.

We can compare *Hura braziliensis* with *Hydrocotyle asiatica,* known in Chinese medicine as Fo-Ti-Tieng. It is a remedy that has been mentioned for leprosy, though in my practice its main use has been in cases of lupus. Being an autoimmune disease, Lupus reflects the self-attacking nature of the mental state. Hydrocotyle is described as a plant with extraordinary rejuvenating effects on the human brain cells and endocrine glands. The herb is found in the marshy, jungle areas of Ceylon, south China, and southwest Asia. Fo-ti-tieng is called 'Elixir of Life' or 'Long Life Elixir.'

Our confusion of orientation, not knowing where we are in the world or where we belong, is an inherent dilemma in evolving cultures. As values are transfused into a greater homogeneity, the distinctions that give one a sense of purpose, are dissolved. The collective becomes the dictator of purpose in society. Values are no longer generated from the revelation or meaning of an inspired culture. Religions become compromised, parables are taught as rules without the underlying initiations. There are fewer moral leaders. The consuming uncertainty of the corporate safety net has us on a course of planned obsolescence in which our lives are the fodder. The working environment becomes narrowed to the point where a computer monitor is the only window to the outer world. Our job descriptions define how we must limit our creativity. This is the disease of homesickness, where we wonder if all these attempts to succeed even bring contentment, let alone joy. We return to our homes at night wondering why we live there.

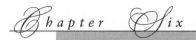

Chapter Six

Treating Anxiety with the Law of Similars

> *Just remember that sickness is the means by which an*
> *organism frees itself of foreign matter, so that one must*
> *just help it to be sick, to have its whole sickness and break*
> *out with it, for that is progress.*
>
> —Rainier Maria Rilke, *Letters to a Young Poet*

[81]

In order to address anxiety we must find where the individual separates the experience of life from its unacceptable disappointments. The resolution of anxiety comes when we can integrate both the conscious and the murky, forgotten fears that we have chosen to suppress over years of defending our lives. Carl Jung based his process of psychological individuation on the alchemical process, which begins with the negredo, the darkness. He described the fundamental beginning process as the integration of the shadow, that we must first address the unacceptable aspects of our personalities before we can move forward.

The medicine in homeopathic work is the shadow. Like Silver, which is used in the making of mirrors, homeopathy finds medicines that reflect our state. The remedy is a meeting with the image of the fear we have been running from. It is our opportunity to turn around and face the fear that is chasing us, thus dissolving its power.

There is a trance induction that begins, "Imagine you are on an island, some place you feel safe. It could be a place in your memory or in your imagination. You must see the colors, smell the smells, and feel the sensations of being there." The importance of this induction is not that such a place exists physically; rather it is that the power of our imagination itself is healing. It begins with our ability to expand our awareness into a larger frame of reference. There is great value in the invocation of sensation-based processing, because sensation is the language of the autonomic nervous system. The imagination has the capacity to create sensory experience. Imagining a visual image would carry less trauma-resolution than imagining the touch of warm sand or smell of fresh air. This is the power of imagination. Our physical body hardly exists beyond our skin, yet our minds are certain of the reality that we have built in defining the world around us. All of us have our own unique world in which we live with certainty and determination. As Proverbs states, "Every man in his own mind thinks he's right, but God looks to the heart."

The island of our imagination is unlimited. The isolated island of our "real world" has more restricted definitions. The egoistic island we live on is dominated by an identification with our personalities. We have developed this island over our whole lives. Like any republic we have defined its borders and secured its defense. Yet any island is surrounded by vast seas and is connected ultimately with the ocean floor and therefore the whole earth.

There is a dream. In the dream we are being chased and can't get away. We try to find some alley or stairwell to escape, but we are helplessly pursued. It is the same in our lives. We may be pursued by expectations or an individual. In terms of finding resolution, it doesn't matter. But when we finally turn around and face our fear it no longer carries the same threat.

In primitive cultures the name of a person or thing carried its potency, its magic, its power. When we define our fear, or turn around and demand, "What is your name, what do you want?" suddenly its potency is dissolved. By naming the bully, the robber, or the oppressor, we then have power over their hidden insecurity of being identified.

We can become too identified with our problems. In one sense naming the problem can bring hidden knowledge to consciousness. This is the positive aspect of diagnosis. By naming a disease or a dysfunction we can then approach it. We need a language to bring to consciousness our experiences, feelings, and fears. On the other hand, excessive identification and attachment to the pathology can maintain its dominance over our lives. When the children of alcoholics are identified with the title of "Adult Child of an Alcoholic," (or the acronym ACOA) it may help them to understand their history. Their difficulties in achieving a successful adulthood may because have its source in unsuccessful parent models. Yet at any age we find those who still blame their parents. An adult is someone who takes responsibility for life; it is no longer projected upon the mother, the father, the world or the stars. It is no longer the government, our teachers, or our spouses who cause our pain and dysfunction. If the explanation for our unhappiness is that the world outside ourselves is to blame, then we have forgotten how to direct our lives. Identification with the name of a diagnosis can make us codependent with our health care providers and create another layer of protection where we become enabled and dependent on the role of the victim.

A profound fear is generated when we find our identities threatened, our failures exposed, our naked wisp of being hanging from a thread like a seed cast upon the wind.

We restrict our lives, limiting the possible opportunities and responses. We're so sure of our duties and responsibilities, our need to be right, we forget that we have cornered ourselves. Anxiety comes from not being able to accept who we are and how we are responsible for our lives.

Our response to fear creates even more fear. We have increased the metabolism and reactivity of our lives. Anxiety is the natural product of a life lived in the future rather than the present, the realm of possibilities rather than the task at hand.

The Medium Is not
the Message

Our reactivity is stimulated by the sounds and rhythms of modern life that impinge on our senses. The daily input of images and information has grown exponentially as part of our modern world, including images that are not only disturbing, but also conflicting.

When we watch action films, our moods are regulated by the music as well as the images. Formulas are applied to media that are known to pull the strings of our emotions. The pace of the film is outside of any real time frame. Relationships are rapidly formed and sex is performed intertwined with acts of violence. These are not the relationships that we experience in our lives.

If most of the relationships we see or fantasize about are based on such superficial contact, we are in deep trouble. If these images were only entertainment, there would probably not be so much damage, but they form deep impressions on our psyches and culture. In fact, our cultural experiences are becoming more limited due to the pervasive influence of corporate mass media as smaller, independent voices become conglomerated.

If through media we are exposed as a voyeuristic act to sexuality in the context of violence and aggression, intimacy in our lives can become associated with violence and aggression. We think we can separate them, yet in our bodies these responses can become confused.

Sexual arousal and capacity for intimacy are expressed in social contexts. Sex hormones, by themselves, do not evoke

[84]

behavior, but, rather, they make it more likely that behavior will occur when the appropriate stimuli are present. Sexual arousal is associated with activity of both the parasympathetic and sympathetic nervous system.

The parasympathetic system governs relaxation and surrender. It allows the erotic responses of arousal. It is the sympathetic system that is responsible for ejaculation and the orgasmic response in men and women. Knowing that fear and anger can become effect sexual feelings, we can try to recognize when emotions unrelated to our capacity for love are influencing our behavior.

Often sex is used as a release for underlying unresolved emotions that have accumulated throughout the day. This runs the risk of using what is an act of intimacy for the resolution of anger and anxiety. While it is a pleasure, it does not deal with our emotions directly any more than violence would effectively resolve anger. Our emotions are not fooled by temporary diversions. They need to be engaged rather than dismissed.

Change comes from becoming more engaged in life. So when we feel angry at the end of the day it is better to resolve these feelings independent of our intimate relationships. The resolution of anger is best enacted either through communication or physical exertion.

Anxiety and depression can inhibit sexual function and desire, triggering a vicious cycle of failure to perform and feelings of inadequacy. Because anxiety, anger, fear, or other defense reactions can activate the sympathetic nervous system, and because this can lead to an inhibition of the parasympathetic nervous system, these emotional states can cause a block or cessation of sexual feelings.

In hypnosis there is a technique of anchoring experiences and their memories through touch. When positive inductions are stated, the body is touched in a pre-established spot, in order to engage these memories in future sessions. In therapy, touch becomes a positive mode in which resolution or positive experiences are set in our bodies.

A negative experience or conflicting messages can be anchored in our bodies as well. Violations of our physical boundaries remain latent in our memories of physical and emotional traumas. Acts of aggression that are confused with intimacy set unconscious defenses. Touch can become a trigger for old memories and silent rejection.

Double Bind Theory, developed by Paul Watzliwick and Gregory Bateson in the 1950s, is one theory of schizophrenia and its causes. Watzliwick and Bateson found that mixed messages that mask the true emotional content of communication had the potential of driving someone to schizophrenia. We are all a little crazy when we are not being real, when we don't say what we really feel, when we hide behind our fears. Imagine a mother who in a sweet voice tells her child, "Johnny, we don't do that do we?" Imagine the frustration instilled in a child who receives the conflicting message of ridicule and disgrace behind his mother's smiling face. This contradictory communication is a recipe for confusion and fear.

Like the theme in the novel *Catch 22,* by Joseph Heller, the Double Bind Theory shows how conflicting double messages result in irresolvable conflict. Another common example of this conflict is the rigidity of bureaucrats. Even when they agree that your situation is unique, they still cannot go outside the rules: "If we did it for you, we'd have to do it for everyone." This is a conflict between truth, at the level of justice, and societal restrictions.

In *The Politics of Experience,* R.D. Laing proposed that insanity is a normal response to an insane society. How else could we organize such disinformation? The rate of psychological adaptation required in modern life has exposed us to a constant reinvention of expectations.

The Storm of Cultural Transitions

The greatest historical parallel to today's rapid cultural change is the transformation that transpired from the Dark Ages to the Renaissance. During the Dark Ages, the Arabic world had maintained an open society toward ideas and learning, while European society remained closed for centuries.

Diet showed the fundamental change in the minds of the society. Since it was difficult to find uncontaminated water, the people of the Dark Ages depended on drinking alcoholic beverages and living in a state of intoxication. They hadn't yet figured out the value of boiling water to kill bacteria. The old monasteries were known for their ale as much as their knowledge. The crusades brought the growth of trade and the introduction of caffeinated teas and coffees, which in turn led to the Enlightenment. Suddenly stimulants were the primary drink rather than depressants. This was a major shift in consciousness, one which supported Renaissance thinking. This was an internal change, embedded in the diet, yet it had an impact that surpassed many external changes of the era.

Stimulants are still the primarily accepted form of drug use in Western society, since they engender productivity and suppress emotions. It is exactly the acceptance of suppressed emotion that generates the simmering of the volcanic fire that produces fear and anxiety. Caffeine can have longer lasting effects on our biorhythms, sleep cycles and sugar metabolism than we might think. Caffeine has been shown to disrupt our ability to go into an alpha state, the brain activity measured as a wave frequency associated with meditation and relaxation, for eight or more hours. Caffeine acts as a heart stimulant, increasing arterial pressure and often producing palpitations. The buzz and agitation are the sought and valued outcome. The effect of this agitation and its ability to mask forgotten stimuli creates anxieties that pervade our modern lives.

[87]

Fear and Trembling

Finding our place in society can become a difficult task when we feel like invading hordes could destroy our lives at any time. Throughout history, and still in much of the underdeveloped world today, these threats are a daily reality. War, famine, and disease are still a personal experience for many populations. Wars are still being fought for economic development.

By the seventeenth century, weapons evolved from the personal grit of hand-to-hand combat to the use of explosives and guns. This increased primary distance of personal contact, reduced a sense of responsibility for acts of violence, and perpetuated fear. In modern times the distance has become even greater. We bomb from the sky and watch mass destruction repeatedly shown on television. We know what "collateral damage" and "acceptable losses" mean even if we do not see the actual events.

In primitive societies, the threat of attack was more immediately physical or projected upon the universe through myth. Abstract fears were caused by gods and goddesses, sacred animals, and totems. Other fears were direct threats, and were engaged instinctually as survival mechanisms. When a jaguar darted from the bushes, the hunter would draw his spear, thrust it into the jaguar's heart, and vanquish his opponent. In the today's world, a modern Jaguar car may approach us with the same degree of threat, yet our response would be limited to honking our horn or swearing at our opponent. We understand why the modern Jaguar poses less of a threat. After all, we are okay, whatever that means to us. Yet our modern internal response is the same as primitive defenses. We carry the effects of this in our body as tension. Lactic acid, adrenaline, and testosterone surge through our systems. Voluntary muscles shorten to strike back and our sympathetic nervous systems prepare for fight or flight.

With little outlet for our tension, we proceed to work. The threat of a car pulling out in front of us is over and perhaps we have even "gotten over it." Then our supervisor comes up to us complaining, "Blah, blah, blah, by two o'clock!" In a primitive society we would have gotten out our spear, thrust it through the supervisor's chest and been promoted. But in today's society we remain passive, afraid of losing a job, and without any true security. By the time we come home, our nervous systems are on fear mode.

The nervous system is divided into two components. One

is the voluntary nervous system. It is expressed through our muscles that voluntarily control movement. The second and more pervasive aspect of the nervous system is involuntary. The involuntary, or autonomic, nervous system regulates respiration, heart rhythm, control of bladder and bowels, and adaptive responses.

If by the end of the end of the workday we have not responded adequately to our stresses, the chemicals of fear in our body accumulate in response to subtle and overt threats throughout the day. Without an adequate physical release, they remain unresolved, building a state of tension in the body.

Then we go home and try to relax. We might have a drink or a smoke. Maybe we have even begun practicing meditation. And while this may resolve our minds, it does not directly impact the capacity of our bodies to discharge this tension. This particular aspect of our embodied fear must be resolved through action. That means we must find some sort of exercise to release our physical tension at the end of the day. Meditation has many extraordinary benefits that have physical results and can help us to become more balanced in our emotional responses but it does not replace movement.

There are two major experiences of anxiety—personal and collective. Collective anxiety arises from our identification with society and its events. Global reporting of instant news, with its emphasis on fear and negativity, creates cultural beliefs based on limited or misinformed perspectives. This is not quite a recommendation for throwing out the television; it's more to raise the point that the mute button may be the greatest invention since the wheel. This collective fear is no different than primitive myth, as it is based on cultural abstractions from our personal experience.

Our own limited perspectives enhance the personal roots of anxiety, which derive from our inability to expand our identities beyond the need to defend and protect ourselves. There are appropriate fears that exist to instinctually protect us, but the overwhelming defenses that we have maintained are mostly antiquated and unnecessary. These anxieties become our pervasive response to threats that no longer exist, but like a car with a

[89]

stuck accelerator, propel us helplessly forward. To address these anxieties requires that we shift the set point, the overactive thermostat that we have set too high, before we suffocate from our own combustion.

HOMEOPATHIC APPROACHES TO ANXIETY

The homeopathic approach to anxiety considers that the regulation of the response is unconscious, even if we know its cause. The solution is not to just eliminate or suppress the signal. Instead we want to trigger the body to reduce or regulate its amperage. Homeopathy as a therapeutic method does not address anxiety at a cognitive level. The explanation from personal history itself does not resolve the inner conflict. We only provide a corresponding reflection of the inner state, through a medicine that mimics it and allows the psyche to self-correct.

The following are a few important examples of how to treat anxiety from the *Homeopathic Materia Medica*. By understanding the clinical pictures of the medicines, we begin to develop a deeper comprehension of the unique situations from which anxiety arises. Our collective experience of healing help us understand how the world of nature reflects our state of mind, helping us to discover and reveal appropriate medicines. The Law of Similars is engaged by recognizing that any substance is capable of effects that mirror the state they can cure.

ACONITE

Aconite is a beautiful and poisonous plant. The flowers are shaped like a monk's hood. Its symmetrical form is suggestive of higher forms of life in the animal kingdom. The higher invertebrates, as well as all vertebrates, possess bilateral symmetry as their fundamental morphological developmental pattern.

Aconite is often mentioned in mythological history. It was supposed to be the principal ingredient in the deadly draught given to the old men of Ceos, when they had become too old to be serviceable to their country. Medea was said to have used it in concocting the poisonous drink she intended for Theseus. It is told that Hecate caused Aconite to spring from the mouth of Cerberus. Theophrastus relates that there was a method of preparing the Aconite so that its action would be delayed, killing its intended victim at the end of one or two years.

The huntsmen of the Alps are said to have dipped their arrows into the juice of this plant when hunting wolves; hence the common name Wolfsbane. In later times it was employed in attempts to destroy whole armies; the Indian poison Bikh or Bisch, with which natives poisoned tanks in the Burmese war, is supposed to have been a prepared from one of its species, *Aconitum ferox.*

As a medicine, the ancients used it chiefly to relieve pain. *Diogenes Laertius* states that the philosopher Aristotle killed himself with a draught of Aconite. The great historian Pliny says it proves fatal when applied to the genital organs of women.

Paradoxically, in Poland, Russia, and Lapland, Aconite was considered harmless, and was used to fatten geese and quails, while some other varieties are said to be eaten as a salad in Sweden.

The classical clinical picture of someone who requires Aconite is extreme restlessness and fear. These people feel they will die from their condition and are so certain of the proximity of their death that they can even predict its imminent approach.

They experience attacks of panic and terror, unreasonable and unaccountable fear, and palpitations. The pathology of someone who requires Aconite can be elicited from a sudden shock or frightening incident, an earthquake, a car accident, or being stuck in an elevator. It can develop into a chronic state of fear. War veterans and police can require Aconite as a result of Posttraumatic Stress Disorder. It is indicated in fears following natural disasters, such as earthquakes, fires and floods. It was the single most important medicine required for survivors in the aftermath of the attack on the World Trade Center in New York City.

The patient requiring Aconite may have fear in crowds or claustrophobia. They will insist on sitting on an aisle seat in a theatre or near an exit. It is useful for women who have the fear of death during pregnancy, especially during labor. The indication for Aconite is recognized by its urgency and immediacy. When it is used in a childhood fever that has come on suddenly, it may also be indicated for the child's caregivers who are fearful and agitated.

SILVER *(Argentum metallicum)*

Mythologically, silver has been associated with the feminine principle and lunacy. The argentums are characterized by phobias and impulsive responses to things, being useful in bringing an uncontrolled imagination into order. Silver, like *Gelsemium sempervirens,* is useful for anxiety before examinations. The main theme is anticipation. Reflecting its capacity to conduct electricity, silver is a medicine for the overactive impulses of the nervous system. Like the silver in photographic film and papers, it helps retain memories, strengthening the coherent organization of the mind.

As the moon relates to water and to the tides, so silver relates to emotional fluxes and periodic cycles. Silver has a significant relation to the female organs, the menstrual cycle, and the ovaries and testes. Reflecting the etymological associations of lunacy and the moon, the womb was associated with causing hysteria. Thus hysterectomy, the removal of the uterus, was a radical yet all too common procedure until recently. There is still a preoccupation in our modern culture with premenstrual syndromes and hormonal fluctuations as an explanation for feminine behavior, rather than an imbalance that may need to be addressed. Silver is one remedy that can bring balance to menstrual cycles.

Silver has an important role to play in the processes of reproduction and gestation. It is used in swelling of the testes and swelling of the urethra in men. In women it is indicated in excessive uterine bleeding, ovarian swelling and pain, especially in young widows or women who have not borne children

The water organs, the kidney and bladder, are also prominently affected in the pathology of Silver. There may be profuse urination, symptoms suggestive of diabetes or pre-diabetic states, and chronic inflammation of the urethra. Silver Nitrate *(Argentum nitricum)* was traditionally used for the treatment of gonorrhea. It has been used as a disinfectant in the eyes of newborns.

Silver in colloidal preparations, suspended particles in minute concentrations, has remarkable antibiotic properties.

Silver is a primary remedy in the treatment of common neurotic states. The patient requiring silver is usually warm-blooded. They are constantly in a hurry, accomplishing little or nothing. They worry about being late when there is plenty of time. They may have suicidal thoughts or irrational impulses that appear suddenly. There can be mental exhaustion from worry, with nervous excitement and trembling. They may pace back and forth or take long walks to discharge their anxieties.

The use of Silver preparations helps to reestablish a rhythmic order between the internal cycles and the surrounding environment. It reduces the state of reactivity that perpetuates senses of anticipation and fear.

CANNABIS

This remedy is prepared from Indian hemp, *Cannabis sativa* or *Cannabis indica,* a hallucinogenic plant that is widely distributed throughout the world, both by natural dispersion of their seeds and commerce. Today marijuana use is one of the most widespread social drugs.

Cannabis is found throughout history. The Ismaili sect contacted by the Crusaders in the eleventh and twelfth centuries were a society known as the Hashishin, Hashish eaters, or the Assassins. The drug was employed to drive cult members to undertake political assassinations, carried out with fanatical ruthlessness and a reckless disregard of death. In modern use, the patient requiring cannabis as a remedy may present in sev-

[93]

eral ways. The themes found in the effects of cannabis are fantasy, theorizing, and amnesia. There is inappropriate laughter and paranoia.

The spacey types of people who might be prescribed Cannabis have a tenuous connection to their bodies and a tendency to feel they are out of their bodies. They may have used a lot of marijuana or other psychedelic drugs in the past.

Cannabis patients can present tremendous belief systems that are not supported by any action in their lives. Like marijuana users, they may associate their experience with spiritual exploration and awareness; however, it is almost a polarity to true spiritual exercise. Cannabis use promotes the dispersal of awareness. This drawing out of the ego that one experiences may in fact seem like a revelation or release of anxiety, but the Cannabis effect is also the enhancer of paranoia and delusional perceptions.

True spiritual experience is based on the focusing of awareness, rather than its dispersion. Cannabis and hallucinogens can produce self-aggrandizing ideations, projecting the experience of enhanced sensory experiences into cosmological fantasies. While the loss of inhibition experienced under hallucinogens may release suppressed emotions or experiences, it is not the replacement for a sustained integration of a transcendent experience. The litmus test for the division between psychosis and mystical experience is our ability to act on it in our daily lives.

This is the central pathology of cannabis; it creates a state in which fantasies can become the guiding experience of life. As the cannabis patient's imagined worldview expands, their ability to ground their emotions and thoughts and function consistently in the world around them is subverted. This separation from society may serve as a verification of the uniqueness of their perceptions. This can be a form of imagination, which gives them a feeling of spiritual inflation.

The reality of spiritual experience can be detected by its ability for the individual to function more creatively and effectively in life. It's grounded in the ability to find happiness in life, rather than in escapist theories.

There is another presentation of the Cannabis type. It is the other polarity of the attempted dissolution of the ego. In fact, Cannabis patients can have very defined ego boundaries. There is a great fear in losing control. The controlled person who requires Cannabis as a medicine appears very similar to the clinical picture requiring *Arsenicum album.*

Arsenicum is one of the main homeopathic medicines used in anxiety states. Arsenicum patients want order in their world to compensate for their fears that something will go wrong. They can be very fastidious and compulsive. They are uptight worriers whose fears and anxieties drive everyone around them crazy. Like Woody Allen, they can be extreme hypochondriacs. They won't go into bathrooms at restaurants because they are worried about contamination and filth. They may have extreme diets or theories about what may cause cancer.

In the controlled type of Cannabis patient we frequently see great anxiety about health and fear of death. These people tend to have avoided marijuana for fear of losing control, or they may have had paranoid and fearful experiences smoking it. Some may feel that they have never been well since a period of marijuana use.

Another hallucinogen used in homeopathic practice is *Agaricus muscarius,* or Amanita, a mushroom that was used by Siberian shamans to induce ecstatic states. The clinical picture of Amanita is similar, with extreme anxiety states and fear of disease, especially cancer.

It is as if the loss of inhibition brings us closer to death-like experiences and the fear of our loss of identity. On the other hand, we may experience a sense of freedom from dissociating from our ego personalities. It is this polarity that is enhanced by the use of cannabis and other hallucinogenic plants. The deep association between the pathological effects of hallucinogenic drugs and their ability to produce both deep anxieties and psychotic experiences leads us to their indications in clinical practice.

This is a clinical picture of patients who require Cannabis as a medicine. It is not meant to judge an individual's use of marijuana or serve as a justification for the incarceration of marijuana users, any more than a clinical description of Tobaccum

[95]

would be. There is no medical justification for such biases or controls. The pathological effects of marijuana elicit the pervasive mental state in which we are trying to escape, to create an idealistic life, rather than engage in the culture at large.

These represent a few of the central themes in the psychological profiles used in the homeopathic treatment of anxiety and panic. By understanding the roots of anxiety and its pathogenesis in the individual we can elicit fundamental changes in behavior and experience.

Chapter Seven

The Immune System: Specific Induction and Non-Specific Resistance

What do we mean by the idea of our immune system? It pervades our every cell. It is the memory of past responses. It represents our boundaries, the recognition of self and non-self. It is autonomic, primitive, and requires no thought. Yet our minds change its course. How we feel alerts or represses immunity. We can enhance the immune system through our states of being, nutrition, and botanical medicines. Yet our immune response is keyed by specificity. It is the language and conformation of geometrical structures within the molecule that trigger a response. It is comparable to two spaceships finding each other and locking in space. We have rhythms within us, biological ebbs and flows of alertness and rest. Different systems are more responsive at different cadences of light and darkness. Biological rhythms awaken different systems at different times. This confirms the observations of Chinese medicine, that the liver is more active before the dawn.

We do not always see the problem that remains unconscious to us. The door may be open but it is the capacity for recognition, the ability to develop flexibility in orientation, that allows us to come and go. Like birds caught in the house, we fly into the windows, having forgotten the door through which we came.

We have mapped the genome and the codes of viruses, yet their primal knowledge is still a mystery, even when their obvious effects can be demonstrated. Our bodies have their own knowledge. It is a symbiotic relationship, an ecology. It is our interaction with the unseen world.

Our immune systems are the boundaries that define our selves. They protect us by allowing nutrients into our bodies, excluding that which is foreign and destructive. There are several components. The primitive immune system consists of natural killer cells and interferons, which patrol our bloodstream stopping the replication of foreign viruses. Our more evolutionarily developed T cells (thymus derived) and B cells (bone marrow derived) act more specifically with the memory of previous infections to attack specific antigens on bacteria and viruses. The focus of immunological research has been on the T and B cells and their activity. The model of our bodies at war against disease is based on the destructive capacities of this part of the system.

However, the more primary aspects of the immune system are those functions that prevent the formation of disease. Our intestines' bacterial flora and immunoglobulins prevent the entry of foreign bacteria and viruses into the bloodstream. Natural killer cells and interferons prevent the replication of viruses. Natural killer cells are capable of spontaneously lysing virus-infected cells and embryonal cells without any evident prior exposure to a specific antigen. Natural killer cells are regulated by interferons and interleukin.

The discovery of interferons led to the understanding of the primitive immune system as a mechanism of non-specific resistance. It was described as the Paul Revere of the immune system that would alert the other cells that the viruses were coming. The mechanism of non-specific resistance controls the minimal pathological drift; its role is not often seen. It discovers the unseen. It is compared to the light of an electrical lamp that cannot be seen in the sunlight. Yet non-specific resistance can be very powerful.

These mechanisms effectively neutralize activated oxygen (free radicals) as well as providing preferential degradation of chemicals and abnormal proteins that can lead to tumor formation and aging processes. The DNA repair system prevents the damage of the genome. The interferon system prevents the disturbance of protein synthesis.

The focus of medical research has been the fighting of bacterial infections. While the knowledge of the specific immunity of antibodies was concurrent with non-specific factors of anti-infectious immunity such as chemotaxis, opsonins, phagocytosis, and complement, the central function of antibodies in infections became the dominating doctrine of research and therapeutics. Because of the efficacy of antibiotics, the strength of endogenous systems were ignored and a predominant dependence on a singular method persists in practice.

Interferon and Non-Specific Resistance

The discovery of interferon initiated tremendous efforts to develop a pharmaceutical agent that could be effective in the treatment of tumors. This led to certain problems because of the bias in American research toward patentable substances. It has been my method to study the original research preceding pharmaceutical research. Pharmaceutical research is too often motivated by profit, ignoring the benefits of nature and natural products. It is often pure science that gives us insights into our greatest, and often disregarded, medicines.

The original discovery of interferon was from the work of Findlay and MacCallum of Great Britain. They found that monkeys infected with Raft Valley Fever Virus were protected from the effects of the more fatal Yellow Fever Virus. Later, Alick

[99]

Issacs discovered that an inactivated flu virus in cell cultures reduced susceptibility to flu viruses. He also discovered that the inactivated virus stimulated what he called "interferon" agents, which prevent viruses from entering other cells and reproducing.

Specific Induction

This is remarkable in light of Samuel Hahnemann's observation of viral interference, published in the *Organon of Medicine* in 1810. Forty years before viruses were described, Hahnemann was observing viral diseases and developing medicines for their treatment. Hahnemann described that a substance that caused reactions similar to a disease state could act as a medicine to stimulate the body's inherent defenses. Hahnemann noted that a disease of a similar nature is capable of eradicating the other rather than becoming compounded in the organism. He gives his examples from the medical literature his time. He describes Edward Jenner's experiences of smallpox eradicating cowpox. It was Jenner who introduced the smallpox vaccine to modern medicine, though there had been earlier examples. He quotes from William Cullen's *Elements of the Practice of Medicine* the account of a measles epidemic in which children were protected from a concurrent whooping cough outbreak. A chronic herpetic eruption was cured by an outbreak of measles. As in our own times, many treatments utilized then were either erroneous or simply detrimental.

However, Hahnemann disagreed with his contemporaries who recommended the use of pathological tissues called nosodes in the treatment of the same disease. This practice, called isopathy, utilizes products of the same disease rather than the similar. It is similar to vaccination, which utilizes disease products in treatment. Unlike vaccination, which is a preventative method, isopathic treatment is used on those who are already sick. Hahnemann said of this practice, "Nothing can come of it but mis-

[100]

fortune and aggravation of the disease." This was not the conclusion of all subsequent homeopaths, however.

Unlike many contemporary homeopaths, Hahnemann makes
only positive responses to the introduction of the smallpox vaccine. The modern problems that have arisen with vaccines are
most likely related to their method of preparation, rather than
any general theoretical flaw to their application. Viral contamination, the types of toxins used to increase immunological
response, and the purity of the individual batches are what have
caused most problems with vaccines.

A related isopathic method used today is that of allergy
desensitization shots, where a diluted preparation of the suspected causative agent is used. The common naturopathic use
of glandular tissues of animal organs and glands to strengthen
their human equivalents is another example.

The use of specific organs and glands is reminiscent of the
Native American practice of eating the heart of the bear for
courage, or Asian fetishes with rhinoceros horns and penises.
There may be some basis for use of such remedies, but in most
cases there are more effective and less problematic approaches.

The doctrine of signatures is a method of finding a substance's use as a medicine based on its sign or form. So a walnut,
based on its shape, may be good for the brain or the intestines.
Chelidonium majus, or Greater Celandine, was found to be a
medicine effective in liver disorders because of its yellow sap
that mimicked the color of bile.

The great medical reformers, Paracelsus and Rademacher
(1772–1850), recommended the use of particular medicines for
the treatment of specific organs. This evolution in prescribing
from the fifteenth through the nineteenth centuries was the basis
for current understandings of diagnosis and treatment.

Hahnemann concluded that the safest and most effective
method of treating diseases was through a medicinal agent that
could mimic the disease. He introduced in his book, *Chronic
Diseases,* published in 1824, forty-eight new remedies for the
treatment of chronic ailments, including what we now know to
be viral diseases. He was particularly interested in the treatment

of the chronic effects of venereal diseases, emphasizing syphilis and gonorrhea. His use of *Thuja occidentalis* in venereal warts (which is caused by human papilloma virus) is one of his great discoveries.

These discoveries of Hahnemann's directly correspond to later discoveries of viral interference. The concept of the vital force in medicine as a self-regulating mechanism is represented in many ways by the functions of our immune systems. It is deeply responsive and connected with our general state of being and its induction is more elegantly generated by specific messages rather than general tonics. In modern terms, this has been termed specific induction of non-specific resistance.

In response to viruses, as well as to such agents as carcinogens and radiation, the normal and pathological responses of a cell are so closely interrelated that only the body's own regulating and protective systems can exercise a selective therapeutic effect. The source for the regulation mechanisms is the cell itself.

Unfortunately, despite these discoveries, allopathic medical interventions have mostly acted as antagonists or inhibitors of these vital intra-cellular systems of regulation. While much of the study of interferon focused on isolating interferon and engineering a method for reintroducing it into the body, a significant core of research, mostly in Sweden and the USSR, was interested in finding substances that induced the natural defenses of the body to produce endogenous, that is internally produced, interferon.

[102]

PHYTOLACCA DECANDRA

Interestingly, one of the most potent of these substances was derived from the plant Pokeweed *(Phytolacca decandra)*. Phytolacca contains vegetable proteins known as lectins. When these lectins contact cell membranes, they can combine to form bridges between cells, causing agglutination. Lectins are natural, plant-based compounds that have the ability to make white blood cells called lymphocytes. This leads to the preferential killing of tumor cells.

Pokeweed mitogens, proteins found in the plant, have been shown to be capable of stimulating the production of an antiviral substance with biological, chemical, and physical properties identical to that of human interferon. Mitogens stimulate cell division in immunocompetent cells and are being used for the study of control mechanisms in cellular division and differentiation.

The use of *Phytolacca decandra* was developed from native indications by Edwin Moses Hale, M.D. (1829–1899). *Phytolacca decandra* is indigenous to North America, where it is common in light, rich, damp soils. It flowers throughout the summer months. This smooth, purplish-stemmed perennial grows to a height of four to ten feet. Its white flowered racemes become lateral and they grow opposite the leaves as the growth proceeds. The fruit is a deep purple, ten-celled berry. Its thick root is sometimes larger than a man's leg in diameter. The leaves should be gathered just prior to the ripening of the berries.

This plant can be found growing in moist ground in nearly all parts of the continent, along hedges, in neglected fields and meadows, and along roadsides. It flowers from July to September. It was known by various other names, including pigeonberry, garget, scoke, coakum, and pocan. The two last names originated with Indian tribes. This species is found not only in the United States but also in the Azores, North Africa, and China. I found it introduced in the garden of my friend Misha Norland in Devon, England. The *Phytolacca icosandra,* a much smaller species, is a native of South America, extending from Rio de Janeiro to Mexico, and is found in some of the West Indian Islands. The *Phytolacca octandra* is found in the West Indies and Mexico, where the berries are used for washing, like soap. These species possess similar properties.

The extremely acrid young shoots are rendered harmless by boiling and are eaten like asparagus. As the plant grows it becomes cathartic as it approaches maturity. It was, in fact, considered among early writers as equal to Ipecac as an emetic, though its use often caused narcotic effects. It was considered the proper cathartic in partial paralysis of the bowel.

Its toxicity is extensive. Vomiting, diarrhea, frontal headache, and sore throat are the most common symptoms observed. Most

importantly, it is documented in historical and current literature to induce tumor formation.

The berries have a popular reputation as a remedy for cancer and rheumatism. John Uri Lloyd (1849–1936), the great
pharmacist of the Eclectic medical tradition, reported its use by
American Indians who used the powdered root as a poultice.
Early settlers described its application to an inflammatory condition of cow's udders called garget. The Pamunkey Indians of
Virginia boiled poke berries to make a remedy for rheumatism.

In Chinese medicine, Phytolacca is described as having *han,*
or cold properties. The clinical indications are in edematous
swellings with abdominal distension and numbness of the throat.

In homeopathic treatment, the psychological state of the
medicine is described as a loss of personal delicacy, disregard-
ing surrounding objects. There is a sense of an entire indifference to life. This can be seen in adolescence, a state of boredom
and indolence, the classic couch potato who falls asleep with
his robe left open exposing himself unconsciously, food left lying
around in disarray. It is compared with *Hyoscyamus niger,* or
Black Hellebore, for its shamelessness and exposure of genitals.
In Hyoscyamus patients, it is more a sense of lewdness and exhi-
bitionism rather than sloth. There is a wonderful term for these
teenagers: "slackers," which expresses their despondent alienation. There is a loathing to waking in the morning, indifference, apathy, and an aversion to work and business. It reflects in
the sluggish lymphatic temperament of the Phytolacca patient.

[104]

These patients are gloomy and irritable. They don't want
to exert their minds. They awaken with disgust for the business
of the day that can progress into a melancholic gloom with indifference to life and even a desire for death. This might not be a
suicidal state. Phytolacca is not suggested as a true suicidal remedy but rather a state in which they are weary of life. Their
response is, "whatever."

The physical indications for Phytolacca are distinct. Dr.
Robert Cooper (1844–1903) confirmed the use of Phytolacca
in breast cancer. Dr. Cooper introduced the idea of giving preparations that he called arborvital remedies in single doses of a
few drops given every four weeks at the wane of the moon.

These preparations were collected from the living plant in order to preserve its life force in the tincture. They were exposed to the sun for twenty-minute increments, each twenty minutes representing successive increases in potency.

This method was the predecessor to the development of flower essences by Edward Bach. In fact, Bach followed Cooper when he worked at the London Homeopathic Hospital as a gastroenterologist. Bach was a contemporary of Cooper's son, Dr. LeHunte Cooper, who continued his father's work in cancer.

Phytolacca is centrally a medicine related to the glands. It is a classical medicine in sore throats, where there is submandibular and cervical gland swelling. Phytolacca was also called the vegetable Mercury, because like mercury it produced and treated glandular swellings. It was also considered a syphilitic remedy, like mercury, in that its symptomology mimicked both the acute and chronic latent conditions related to syphilis.

Because of the presence of Caustic potash, or Potassium, in Phytolacca, early writers compared its action to Causticum, which is used in homeopathy for conditions affecting ligamentous and connective tissue such as fibromyalgia. Phytolacca patients present with extreme stiffness in all the limbs with fatigue and weakness. They are better from cold baths and worse from deep pressure. These are not cases that are helped by deep bodywork, which only aggravates the Phytolacca patient.

These characteristics distinguish Phytolacca from *Bryonia alba,* or Wild Hops, which is worse for movement and better for deep pressure, and *Rhus toxidendron,* or poison ivy, which is used in patients who are better with movement and worse in a damp climate. Phytolacca patients' pains appear suddenly and disappear suddenly. They are like electric shocks, radiating all over the body. I have seen its efficacy in cases of fibromyalgia, chronic fatigue, and Lyme's disease, where systemic rheumatic pain and fatigue are common.

The attacks of extreme fatigue can be also found in *Ferrum metallicum,* or Iron, which in mythology and astrology is associated with the planet Mars. Like Mars, the patient requiring homeopathic Iron is a warrior. I have found its use particularly helpful for professional athletes who have suddenly collapsed

[105]

and are unable to continue their exercise. Often in these cases, we see young adults who have competed for their fathers' approval as a factor in their competitive exertions.

The example of *Phytolacca decandra* as an immune stimulant, specific to viral conditions and tumors, shows us how the homeopathic method might be a more direct source for developing new treatments, perhaps superior to the more traditional methods of screening medicines in cell cultures for their effects on isolated disease agents. Incorporating an understanding of a medicine's action with its full range of toxicology broadens our understanding of its action. Selectively applying mild doses of what might be toxic substances helps eliminate the current bane of what is relegated as side effects.

This is the future of medicine. We will utilize the fulcrums of the body rather than hammering away at the structure. We will listen for the simple entrance to the problem. The body relies on elegant and sophisticated feedback mechanisms. The body relies on the mirror of self-recognition to respond. What we see in the mirror is not ourselves, it is only an image to remind us of ourselves.

Chapter Eight

From the Womb to the Tomb: A General Theory of AIDS and Cancer

One of the great mysteries in life is contained in its conception. The capacity for the union of sperm and egg is protected by the function of one fundamental hormone, Human Chorionic Gonadotropin, or HCG. The placenta richly produces HCG during pregnancy. The placenta is the tissue or organ formed during gestation through which the mother's blood and nutrition is transferred to the fetus. It is the barrier that protects the fetus from infections present in the mother.

The family of glycoproteins to which HCG belongs is not a recent evolutionary development. Similar proteins have been found in mammals and insects going back to the origins of life. HCG-like proteins have been isolated in bacteria and yeasts such as *Candida albicans*.

Normally, foreign chromosomes are rejected by the body's defenses. Even as a single cell, the union of the parent's chromosomes could be considered as a foreign invading body, much like any foreign bacteria or virus. HCG veils the newly implanted embryo from being rejected as foreign by the mother's body. It is therefore known as the hormone of pregnancy.

HCG also protects the aggressive spermatozoon as they make their journey toward the egg so that the female's immune system will not be able to reject the sperm as foreign invaders.

HCG is found in every cell throughout the body. It is found in sperm and egg. It is produced in small quantities in pulsations by the pituitary gland in the brain. Its highly negatively charged surface makes it immunologically inert. Normal immune system cells from the body cannot destroy it.

Common Threads of Fertility, Conception, Disease, and Death

Ironically, HCG is found in every tumor and cancer cell. It is not the cause of cancer, but it is activated when malignant transformation occurs. HCG protects the cancer cell from being recognized or attacked by the immune system. This is why tumor formation is so insidiously proliferated, undetected until the growth is so great that it interrupts function in some neighboring structure. By the time cancer is detected clinically, it has usually been forming for some time. The presence of HCG also masks the metastatic dissemination of cancer cells.

In an almost cosmological paradox, it has been observed that the growth of the placenta and its regulation by HCG is an embryological model of the growth and regulation of cancer cells. HCG simultaneously protects the growth of the embryo and may contribute to the death of the organism. The embryo and the cancer may also contain the secrets of immortality with their capacity for growing continuously while deriving their nutrition from external sources, compromising the well-being of the host. They do not live symbiotically, Symbiosis means both benefit. However, tumors provide no benefit and are more parasitic in nature. The fetus, on the other hand, contributes to the survival of the mother's species. Fortunately for the mother, the child is born. Unfortunately for the cancer patient, the devouring nature of the cancer undermines the survival of the organism.

In 1902, the Scottish embryologist John Beard noticed the relationship between the growth of the trophoblastic cells that surround a fertilized egg and cancer cells. These trophoblasts attach to the uterus forming the chorionic villi that are the fetus's portion of the placenta. The rapid division, growth, and invasive action of the trophoblasts and placenta were recognized as being correlates for the behavior of cancer. In fact, current methods of treating cancer by stopping the process of angiogenesis (growth of the tumor into surrounding tissue) originate in Beard's discovery. Unfortunately, this method does not address the metastatic potential of cancer.

The placenta does not continue to grow into the wall of the abdomen. Its growth is held in check. Beard proposed that the invasive growth of the placenta into the uterus was stopped in the seventh week at the same time as the first production of pancreatic enzymes by the fetus. The developing embryo does not really need a pancreas to produce insulin for the metabolism of sugars, as adequate levels are provided by the mother. Nor does the fetus need the digestive enzymes produced by the pancreas; it gets all its nutrition maternally.

Yet Beard observed the pancreas produced significant amounts of pancreatic enzymes long before birth. He also studied the microscopic forms of placental and cancer cells both of which appeared undifferentiated. Most normal cells have a definite morphological structure with distinctive internal properties. Cancer and placental cells look more like primitive cells, such as amoeba or simple blobs of protoplasm.

Beard therefore recommended the use of pancreatic enzymes in the form of injections. He published his theories in 1902 in the medical journal, the *Lancet*, and in his book, *The Enzymatic Treatment of Cancer and Its Scientific Basis*. However, others were unable to reproduce his results, a failure Beard attributed to the use of poor preparations or inadequate dosage.

Beard's theories have been resurrected several times in the

alternative cancer treatment movement. Both Ernst T. Krebs and William Kelley based their cancer treatment methods on the use of pancreatic enzymes.

Demonstrating a new approach in 1972, Valentin I. Govallo M.D., Ph.D., and Director of the Laboratory of Immunology in Moscow, published *The Immunology of Pregnancy and Cancer*. In his book, he describes his use of extract of the human chorionic villi from the placenta combined with white blood cells to immunize the patient against the placenta-like cancer. He compares this with other methods of immunotherapy in which he specifically attempted to induce immunoglobulin and natural killer cell responses. The use of placental extracts that he calls immunoembryotherapy has had remarkable success.

Govallo reports that out of thirty-five patients treated, 88.6 percent survived for up to three years, 77.1 percent survived for five years, and 65.4 percent survived for ten years or more. This was in a wide variety of cancers, including breast, lung, uterine, and kidney.

FERTILITY

Since HCG is the hormone that maintains the viability of the fetus, it would seem logical that stopping the production of HCG would lead to infertility. In 1981, Dr. Vern Stevens and his associates at the Department of Obstetrics and Gynecology, Ohio State University, published their paper on a vaccine that attacked HCG.

[110]

This vaccine has proven to be an effective method for birth control for a three-month period with no adverse reactions. The antibody response declines with time. Fertility was regained when concentrations fell. This has remarkable implications for women. The World Health Organization is now in charge of studying this method of birth control.

ANTI-CANCER VACCINES

By attacking the HCG in the membrane of cancer cells, the anti-conception vaccine was also found to be effective in cancer. Hernan Acevedo, Ph.D., et al. did the first experimental studies.

Phase one clinical trials began in 1994, with promising results. Dr. Acevedo is a retired professor of pathology and laboratory medicine at Allegheny General Hospital in Pittsburgh, Pennsylvania. The vaccine has been shown to be effective in colon, pancreatic, lung, and liver cancers. Most importantly, it works on metastatic cells throughout the body.

PREVENTING CANCER IN WOMEN

One beauty of using the HCG vaccine as a method of fertility control is that it should effectively prevent the formation of cancer in women who are using it. Since it does not affect the feedback mechanisms of estrogen, it would not contribute to systemic effects commonly associated with birth control pills.

AIDS and the Antiviral Effects of HCG

Until now we have mainly discussed the effects of attacking HCG to stop its protection of fetal cells and cancer. We must remember, however, that HCG in the developing fetus has an additional effect of being one of the main antiviral components in the embryological immune system.

An infected mother's HIV does not transmit to the fetus due to the presence of HCG. The infection of the fetus occurs when it passes through the vaginal canal and is exposed to the maternal blood. The placental barrier through which the maternal blood passes to the developing fetus in utero is protected by the presence of HCG. In 1992, A.S. Bourinbaiar and R. Nagorny, working at the Population Council for Medical Research in New York, investigated the effects of HCG in cell cultures of viruses including HIV. There was no doubt that HCG was effective against all RNA viruses, including HIV.

In 1995, Robert Gallo at the National Cancer Institute found that HCG inhibited Kaposi's sarcoma.

Working independently at the same time, Pamela Harris

reported her studies of HCG in the treatment of Kaposi's sarcoma in extremely high doses of 150,000 to 700,000 international units, three times per week, with marked tumor regression. However, the costs of such high doses would be economically unreasonable. The work was left unfinished.

In 1998, I attended a conference on Comprehensive Cancer Care in Washington, D.C. and had the privilege of hearing Dr. Acevedo speak on his work with the cancer vaccine that disrupted HCG.

A year later he suggested to me that the same delivery system he had used in the cancer vaccine might be applicable in increasing the absorption of HCG in treating AIDS. This delivery system consists of simple pharmaceutical agents that are used in cosmetics and in injections to increase absorption. It was simple, but remarkable.

Initial responses have showed us that the combination of HCG with adequate absorption could decrease the cost of treatment to an affordable level with remarkable success. While the promise of HCG in AIDS has not been fully studied, our initial clinical experience has shown immediate and astonishing results. It will remain for further studies to demonstrate its efficacy in AIDS and other epidemic viral diseases.

The biological importance of HCG led me to conduct a study of its homeopathic effects. In September 2001, Peter Glidden, N.D. and myself conducted a proving of a 30x potency of HCG in a double blind crossover study of eighteen persons. It is a combination of both the homeopathic provings and information derived from scientific research that creates a more wide ranging understanding of a substance's complexity of effects. While some of the most important symptoms in homeopathic prescribing come from their effects on healthy persons, it is also their known physiological effects which can contribute to a synthesis of pharmacological knowledge. It must be remembered that homeopathic principles are inclusive of toxicological and physiological effects that are capable of enhancing self-regulation in the body rather than being used solely to control physiology. This is an opportunity to see where disregarded effects of drugs may actually contribute to understanding a broader range of their application.

I may have thought because of the physical significance of HCG that it would have produced more pathological features in the experiment. In fact, the preponderance of symptoms were expressed in mental and emotional states.

The overarching sense this proving generated was one of a psychological house cleaning. It was not a pleasant experience for the majority who participated. Old failures would be remembered, one after the next, like scenes in a movie. Provers felt unable to reach destinations, unable to accomplish tasks. These experiences, rather than emotionally purging, left the provers with no relief.

There was a sense of hypersensitivity, as if all their emotions were brought to the surface. Impatience was both a symptom produced by the proving and a cured symptom in one individual who was impatient in general previous to the proving. The proving cured a syndrome of fatigue and muscle tension of the jaw and spine in anther person.

The dreams were of impatience and regrets. There were dreams of not being heard or judged inadequate. They felt they could not reach their destination or were blocked.

One prover dreamt of a visitation by four women angels in which she felt powerful with a sense of peace. They stood in a pentagonal circle with her. Her daily problems which had been plaguing her, vanished after waking. She said she had very few dreams in her life in which good things happened. Another suddenly felt she would like to have another child though she had not wanted more children previously. This would very much seem like an appropriate experience with Human Chorionic Gonadotropin. There is a great enrichment that comes from multidisciplinary studies of medicine. No singular specialty can conclude its findings without a consideration of other fields of study. As we continue our studies of HCG and its profound nature, it will no doubt touch on some of our most primordial experiences as well as our most modern of diseases.

Chapter Nine

Beaten Paths in the Valley of Forgotten Horizons

While a saint operates directly by mean's of God's grace, the physician operates by means of God's Creation ... Nature.

—Paracelsus

[115]

Vitalism is the recognition of the life force as the organizing substratum of material form. It is a philosophy that views our existence as having purpose and direction. Vitalistic philosophy recognizes that there is a larger viewpoint that we believe in, for which inductive proof is generated by the natural observations of its effects. Vitalism is the mystery that differentiates mechanical from organic processes. Organic in chemical language means the organizing materials of life forms. While most life processes are described through the energetics of chemical interactions (enzyme systems, nutrition, etc.), the underlying patterns and forces that generate and organize life processes have been a philosophical as well as theological question that has challenged science. Since many scientists do not believe in God, it is harder to find a scientific model that incorporates the ideas of a life force or spirit. The spiritual or metaphysical remains relegated to the unknowable and unquestioned by science and medicine in general. Vitalism was dismissed as a science simply because there was not an adequate description for it. Yet it has remained the primary philosophy of many of our greatest scientists.

This book is not an attempt to draw conclusions on the scientific validity of vitalism. It is descriptive rather than conclusive. The many tomes on the shelf called the science of this or that can adequately give an explanation for our science. Many of them will also become obsolete as we reach greater understanding. I am more interested in principles that generate a deeper effect of healing.

The abstraction of mathematics is one form for scientific analysis. This is an example of deductive science. Deductive methods reduce the variables to where they can be analyzed. Empirical science is confirmed by experience, whether the explanation is proven or not. Textbooks are written on gravity and its results, but no one knows what gravity is. Even greater works are written on consciousness and spirit, yet it remains through faith that its greatest experience is revealed. These experiences do not fit the rationalist model, being measured through effects rather than pure materiality.

The idea of a vitalistic science is an attempt to direct scientific inquiry and discovery toward the fulfillment of God's creation rather than against it. There is an ethic involved as a guiding principle. These principles emphasize the ability for the healing power of nature to achieve restoration through modeling nature's own intelligence. Knowledge of a vitalistic perspective not only includes the value of deductive thinking, it places it into a context of values that respect the perceived intentions of a greater will. By placing science in the context of the mystery of life, vitalism puts the implications of its effect on the world at large above the ambition of individuals.

This may seem paradoxical. Wars have been fought in the

name of truth. While truth is subject to more than beliefs, observations are not solely proven by linear deductions either. Inductive and empirical reasoning achieve understanding from pure observations of relationships. Vitalistic practice seeks to understand the soil and inner state from which disease arises, not in the causalistic sense, but as a relationship. The vitalistic is expressed through an ecological awareness and seeks understanding through patterns. It is respectful of the consequences of actions. Vitalistic approaches make different assumptions. Life is always a miracle, despite our explanations. More happens in healing from what we don't know than what we do.

Vis Medicatrix Naturae: The Healing Power of Nature

The Western tradition is older than Greek civilization, but Greek thought represents a central turning point in describing the forces that have created our modern medical philosophy and practice. With the exception of certain Egyptian texts, the first descriptive analysis of disease was the works ascribed to Hippocrates. Hippocrates was born around 460 B.C. on the island of Cos; he died around 370 B.C.

Hippocrates taught the empirical method, that each person's disease was individual. He saw that classifications of disease and symptoms were theoretical; therefore, treatment was based on the characteristics of the person. Details of their life and behavior were considered essential. "Speech, manners, fashion, even his silence, his thoughts ... the content and origin of his dreams ... one has to study all of these signs and to analyze what they portend." Physical diagnosis was primary. The odors, excretions, and physical appearance were important. Probes and speculums were introduced to examine orifices and genitalia.

The roots of the conflict between materialistic science and vitalism were already evident in the Hippocratic writings. These

[117]

writings were actually the works of several authors, some supporting treatment by contraries through the humoral theory. The primary humors were hot, cold, dry, and moist. The treatments that balanced the humors were opposite to the nature of the disease. A hot disease would be treated by cooling herbs and baths.

This led to the development of the allopathic approach, even to the practice of bloodletting and salivation with mercury to balance the body. The body fluids were made of blood, phlegm, and yellow and black bile. Excess or deficiency of these fluids led to disease. The resolution or therapeutic reaction to disease was fever or coction, that is a "boiling" with a discharge of the excessive bodily humor or fluids. In this method, the crisis was the source of healing. The way to achieve this was disputed.

Other writings in the Hippocratic corpus, particularly *Ancient Medicine and The Art,* emphasized the Law of Similars, which represents the use of medicinal and symbolic methods which stimulate the healing power of nature. Writings based on a rationalistic theory attempts to find which treatment will be most effective in manipulating physiology, while the other seeks to arouse the inherent passages toward healing.

The empirical method utilizing the Law of Similars, would also introduce hygiene, dream analysis, and predecessors to our modern hypnosis and psychology.

Another aspect of the humoral theory was one of constitutional types. It was through this aspect of the humoral theory that both methods could approach the body as a whole. The constitutional types were physical structures and emotional states which dominated the characteristics of the individual. The four types described are sanguine, choleric, phlegmatic, and melancholic.

The sanguine person is a jovial extrovert. They respond to others openly. They tend to get caught up in drama, often being overly sympathetic. They are optimistic and loving, yet often they are seen as superficial and difficult to depend on. However, they are as easily loved as forgiven. They are "happy without direction."

The choleric person is also extroverted, but not so sympathetic. They are vital and energetic, yet demanding and forceful. They are "hot-headed," angry, and critical when they don't get their way. Their strength also lies in their magnetic natures. They are the spark that ignites the fire. The strength of their personality can draw others toward their plans and success. They view the world as a battle to be won, forcing their will to achieve their goals.

Phlegmatic people are more down to earth. They appear kind, reliable, and trustworthy. They are calm and able to reflect and make pragmatic decisions in the midst of a storm. They can be the pillars of strength. Their desires can be very material, yet this is the type that can often be the most accurate in their intuition.

Melancholics are more introverted. Their feeling is held inside. Often they feel jaded, having soured on life. They are hurt easily and hold grudges silently or for long periods of time. They are pessimistic. However their depressive nature is not all negative. M. Esther Harding wrote a wonderful article called, "The Value of Depression," in which she describes how these deep states of depression are in many ways characteristic of the most creative and spiritual people. Depression allows us the full depth of emotional experience if we don't get caught in it.

Humours can be viewed like modern physiology through the eyes of its mechanism or dynamics. These constitutional humoral types allow us to understand the dynamic expression of the physical state.

The Greeks were among the first to attempt a model of disease that did not see illness as a punishment of the gods or a curse. Of course, magical medicine was still a respected part of Greek medicine. Yet the fundamental direction of philosophic and scientific inquiry was influenced by Plato and the Dogmatists. They based their ideas on logic. However, in logic, assumptions upon which you reach conclusions have to be accurate as well. The often faulty speculations that were the basis for their logical assumptions came without direct experimentation for confirmation. These inaccuracies led to extreme treatments attempting to balance humors or arouse coction, consisting of bleeding and purging, and these continued to be practiced into the nineteenth century.

After Hippocrates, Rome influenced the course of medicine. The allopathic approach was represented by Galen. Although his philosophy was vitalistic, his therapeutic approach was largely rationalist and became the basis for treatment for the next 1,500 years, through the Dark Ages. His tremendous observations of anatomy were mostly based on animals and therefore were not always accurate in human terms. However, his clinical observations were unequalled in his time. His treatments were generally Hippocratic in nature, involving functional treatments such as we have in modern naturopathic practice. He was known for combining large numbers of plants, referred to as Galenicals. This polypharmacy has persisted in herbalism to this day. The modern herbal and nutritional industry has become a force for the use of wide ranging substances with general benefit, exemplifying a Galenic approach. Galen developed a medicine called Theriac, originally intended against snake venoms, which came to be used as a universal antidote for all poisons and infectious diseases. In Galen's time, the contents of Theriac increased beyond seventy substances, and by the Middle Ages over a hundred medicines could comprise its recipe.

The Renaissance of Medicine

Throughout the Middle Ages, the use of wide ranging treatments based on opposition of humors superseded careful investigations of the causes of disease, failing to recognize infections or hygiene sources. Physical diagnosis was limited and anatomical information was mostly inaccurate. New ideas were considered heretical. Medical teachings referred back to Galen, whose authority had become fossilized. His certainty of success in treatment, combined with a vitalistic Hippocratic philosophy that the Church could approve, assured his dominance in medical matters where few translations or resources were available.

It was not until the sixteenth and seventeenth centuries that these ideas were challenged. From the therapeutic perspective, Paracelsus introduced a revolution in chemistry and medicine that pervades the whole premise of this book. From an anatomical perspective, Vesalius introduced dissection and the mapping of the body, dispelling the speculations of Galen.

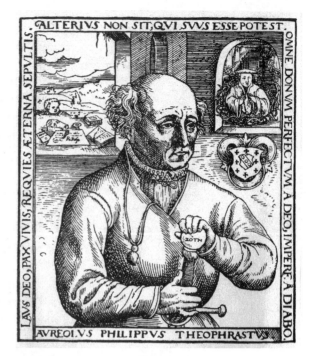

Paracelsus was a traveling physician who took his knowledge from every walk of life. He worked in mines, extracting knowledge of the use of metals and minerals in medicine. He studied alchemy in the laboratory of Sigismund Fugger. He shared the teachings of the occult philosopher Johannes Trithemius with his contemporary Cornelius Agrippa. However, Paracelsus sur-

Paracelsus

passed his contemporaries in that he applied his theoretical cosmology and Christian theology to the applications of medicines, testing them in the fire of human suffering. These powerful medicines became the center of a controversy that persisted in England and France for two centuries. He introduced the use of chemical medicines, not in their crude form, but in refined preparations based upon alchemical practice. Paracelsus maintained that any poison had medicinal properties depending on its proper preparation and dosage. In particular, his introduction of minute quantities of mercury for syphilis threatened not only the medical societies, but also the merchant class that imported the plant Guaicum from Haiti for its treatment.

He maintained the Doctrine of Signatures as a morphological basis for determining a substance's indications in disease. He produced medicinal quintessences that refined poisons to extract their virtue or "Arcanum." Man was seen as part of nature, as the corresponding function of stars on earth.

Paracelsus challenged the medical establishment. He eventually earned a temporary teaching position in Basel, where he taught in the common Swiss German of the times rather than the conventional Latin. His first lecture was on the importance of the fires of digestion, for which he has been acknowledged as the originator of biochemistry. He burned the writings of Galen and Avicenna on midsummer's night to protest their authority, which led to the protests of his colleagues and his subsequent dismissal.

Paracelsus traveled throughout Europe at a critical time in history. This was the time of Martin Luther and the Humanists. Paracelsus treated Erasmus and was physician to the Teutonic Knights. An apocryphal story tells that he was captured in Russia by the Tatars, Mongolian tribes who raided villages and towns. His life was spared because of his tremendous medical and surgical skills that were used on the battlefields. He himself was fascinated by the Tartars' shamanistic practices, faith healing, and use of physiognomy, the reading of facial features.

Paracelsus's influence is felt throughout medicine. He was, however, representative of the chemistry of his times. Natural science was seen as the expression of religion. There was no division. His four pillars of medicine were natural philosophy, astronomy, alchemy or chemistry, and virtue or righteousness. He was unique in the strength of his writings and he was renown for his cures, particularly in the difficult diseases such as gout, leprosy, and epilepsy.

Paracelsus had few students during his lifetime. The Paracelsian physicians arose thirty or more years after his death. Joan Baptista Van Helmont, who discovered gases, was an avid Paracelsian. By the eighteenth century, much of Paracelsian philosophy was dismissed in the rise of mechanistic principles. Samuel Hahnemann, who introduced homeopathy, does not mention Paracelsus in his writings, though he is one of the more modern exponents of his principles. Constantine Hering, who developed homeopathy in the United States, maintained a library devoted to the writings of Paracelsus. Spagyric and Anthroposophical medicines are based on many of his ideas, and while they represent a minority of medical practitioners, they persist to this day. Although much of his writings seem steeped in the occultism and natural magic of his times, these doctrines were not the black magic we think of today but a natural science that was largely inspired in the accepted doctrinal context of the Church.

Paracelsus saw salt, mercury, and sulfur as representing inner qualities as well as elements. His world was still participatory; it engaged the elements as chemical representations of our inner processes as well as cosmological events. Through engaging these universal substances found in nature, one could come to understand the development of the universe itself and become an active participant in the creative process of the world.

The Life Force

The archeus or life force of Paracelsus was the basis for subsequent models of a vitalistic source toward understanding human health and disease. The introduction of the concept of anima by Georg Ernst Stahl (1660–1734) was the basis for vitalistic theory in the eighteenth century. Like the "physis" of Hippocrates and the "psyche" of Aristotle, Stahl rejected the reductionist movement of mechanical science. Yet Stahl still maintained a strong support for bloodletting to reduce "plethora." Although his philosophy represented the foundation for vitalistic philosophy of his times, he maintained allopathic approaches to treatment. Bloodletting was based on the idea that it would relieve excessive heat in the system to balance the humors.

Stahl was succeeded by French physician Paul Joseph Barthez (1734–1806). For a time, Barthez was a consulting physician to the King. He referred to the "Principle of Life." After 1773, the term vitalism came into general use. He saw this force as separate from the soul, a unifying principle of organ systems that was modified by their function. The outward material form was determined by the expression of an inner force. These concepts were developed at a time when William Harvey's Circulation of the Blood supported Rene Descartes's views that the body was simply a machine. Descartes also postulated the pineal gland as the location of the soul in the brain, a divergence from his other, often materialistic, thoughts.

In the late eighteenth and nineteenth century, the leading representatives of vitalistic medicine were Hahnemann and Anton Mesmer.

Anton Mesmer (1734–1815) is best known today for his introduction of suggestive trance induction, which became known as mesmerism, or hypnosis. Mesmer was experimenting with the use of magnets and the transmission of healing forces in treatment. His descriptions of "animal magnetism" followed Paracelsus's ideas of a universal principle that could be transmitted, and paralleled Galvini's demonstration of the action of electricity at a distance. Mesmer became extremely popular among the French aristocracy. His charismatic group treatments in his salon included tubs in which animal magnetism could be transferred to ailing parts of the body. These were accompanied by the eruption of emotional crises as the purported results of releasing obstructed animal magnetism. Mesmer was in many ways the predecessor to modern body psychotherapies in addition to his emerging concepts of healing energies. Unfortunately, Mesmer was not popular with his scientific contemporaries. At the behest of the Royal Society, King Louis XVI was persuaded to form a commission that condemned Mesmer and refused him the right to practice medicine. Mesmer's career was a short, controversial flame, which he was content to leave behind him in retirement.

Organicism

Johann Wolfgang von Goethe (1749–1832) was among the first to use the term morphology. Morphology is the study of underlying form, the intimate relationship between shape and structure and the processes governing function. The relationships of the conformation of structures to their biological function, whether on the cell membrane, plant forms, or in visual images, is the basis for the doctrine of signatures.

The eighteenth century became the turning point for the controversies and increasing division between mechanism and vitalism. The persistent interrelationship of these seemingly opposing ideas continued to evolve.

In chemistry, it was discovered that substances with the same chemical components could act differently based on their geometrical configuration. In 1826, Wohler and Liebig observed cyanic and fulminic acid had the same composition and structure, but different geometric orientations. This led to the discovery of isomerism. Isomerism described how the direction in which light was refracted through a compound differentiated its function from identical chemicals of the same composition.

In biology, the "field" is the most important concept dealing with underlying patterns as an organizing principle. Alexander Gurwitsch first used the term in 1922. The embryologist, Paul Weiss, used field concepts in 1926 to explain limb regeneration in amphibians. We know how each of our fingerprints is unique, and if we are cut, we heal with the same pattern. But we don't know how the genome acts to orchestrate such unique characteristics. We know that when a limb is cut off, there can still be sensation of that extremity. The brain is capable of reorganizing to compensate for misinformation.

Weiss developed the concepts of Organicism with his colleagues Ross Harrison and Joseph Needham. Needham went on to become one of the world's leading sinologists culminating in his epic work, *Science and Civilization in China*. I mention this because of his profound description of Chinese systems of energetics that forms the basis of their practices of medicine and alchemy.

Yet Harrison and Needham's goals in describing the phenomenon of embryological development were to find a purely chemical explanation. Organicism became the field for attempting to characterize vitalistic phenomena in mechanistic terms. We are given the intersecting points, which define a new course for understanding the different lenses through which life can be observed. Organicists believed that life was self-generating solely from the mechanisms within the cell and organism. Nutrition provided the necessary energetic sources. There was no soul-infusing life.

The open systems theory of Ludwig von Bertanalaffy postulated in the 1940s that living systems are open to and interact with their environments. He described how these systems could acquire qualitatively new properties through emergence, which is a process of continual evolution. He saw biological systems as maintaining equilibrium outside of the laws of thermodynamics and physics.

The concepts of neurological function became the context within which a description of vitalism was debated. Attempts to describe nerve impulses in terms of electrical or magnetic forces were considered inadequate. It was the demonstration of the chemical basis for nerve impulse transmission in 1921 by the physiologist Otto Lowei, which defined modern neurophysiology. It is reported that Lowei had repeated dreams in which the method for the experiment was shown to him.

It was assumed that the triumph of chemical and mechanistic demonstrations of nerve impulses in physiology eradicated the remaining postulations of vitalism.

However, Robert Becker's work with salamanders showed that the organizing factor of limb regeneration and healing was in fact electrical and electromagnetic in nature. He showed that it was perineural Schwann cells that carry electrical signals that cause fractures to heal, not the nerves!

The standard concepts of immunology are changing as well. Conventionally known forms of intercellular communication involving the lock and key concept of antibody and antigen interaction in immunology, or ligand-receptor interactions, are slow processes over short distances. But cells also need rapid communication over long distances. It is postulated that cell membranes are an amplification site for weak electromagnetic fields capable of stimulating or suppressing many cell functions.

We now know that magnetic fields are generated from the pineal gland and influence circadian cycles or biorhythms. The pineal gland regulates all other glands of the body, producing melatonin, serotonin, and dopamine that regulate brain function. It has been shown that the pineal gland responds to changes in the Earth's magnetic field, despite the weakness of the field's force. The pineal also regulates our biological clock, a key substrate of autonomic function.

I remember in ninth grade biology when we were shown images of mitosis and meiosis, the division of cells, I always wondered what the lines connecting the movement of the cells were. I later found these were magnetic fields.

We know we are mostly water. Like the tides, our bodies are influenced by the cycles of the earth and moon. Solar magnetic field activities have twenty-two-year cycles affecting patterns in human affairs. Perhaps there are other subtle effects from other gravitational fields, magnetic storms and celestial events that though slight when compared to the direct biological effects impacting us, have more long-range influences. These would confirm Paracelsus's belief that we are microcosmic expressions of the greater patterns in our universe.

> Of late I have attempted to look into the problems furnished by nature, rather than those more superficial ones for which our artificial state of society is responsible.
>
> —Sherlock Holmes, just before his death in
> *The Final Problem*

Resonance: The Affairs of the Heart

If you isolate a cell from the heart, keep it alive, and look at it through a microscope, you will see it lose its rhythm and begin to fibrillate until it dies. If the heart cell is put in close proximity to another cell, it will synchronize rhythms and beat in unison. Without touching they communicate across a spatial barrier. This union is demonstrated between two people whose emotional relationship shares information. These phenomena are obviously difficult to explain in simple linear terms. Spontaneously rhythmic mechanisms, known as "oscillators," can be expected to lock onto a nearby strong enough rhythmic influence. Paradoxically, the heartbeat can be accelerated by an inhibitory stimulus, made to cycle faster by more frequent inhibition, and slowed down by the increasing rate of stimuli that individually accelerate it.

PARADOXES OF PHARMACY

This is reminiscent of a principle in pharmacology that underlies homeopathy and hormesis. Hormesis is the study of low dose effects of toxins. The Arndt-Schultz Law describes the paradoxical inverse relationship of low dose toxins having greater physiological stimuli. This is known as a drug's biphasic action. Normal doses of atropine, which is derived from the plant Belladonna, block parasympathetic nerves, causing mucous membranes to dry up, while minute doses can cause increased secretions of mucous membranes.

Weak stimuli *accelerate* physiological activity. Medium doses *inhibit* activity, and large doses are toxic.

In physiology, Wilder's Law of Initial Value states that the greater the initial stimulus, the *smaller* the change or response. Medium ranges of stimuli affect a greater tendency toward absent and frequently reversed or paradoxical responses. The higher these extreme initial stimuli, the more frequent the reversals on function raising stimuli. The lower the initial stimuli the more frequent are the reversals on function depressing stimuli. These paradoxes explain why animals or humans do not have identical responses to identical stimuli, such as medications.

In genetics, our understanding of the role of DNA is more dynamic and less linear. While the overwhelming concepts of biology are founded on the unalterable effects of DNA, the traditional paradigm of a gene coding for a protein and subsequently a specific phenotype, has been realized to be too simplistic.

A genotype is the internally coded, inheritable information or blueprint carried by all living organisms. They are copied at the time of cell division or reproduction and are passed from one generation to the next. A phenotype is the outward, physical manifestation of the organism. These are the physical parts, the sum of the atoms, molecules, macromolecules, cells, structures, metabolism, energy utilization, tissues, organs, reflexes, and behaviors; anything that is part of the observable structure, function, or behavior of a living organism. So the genotype codes for the phenotype. This is the genetic code.

Genes are influenced by both the genetic and external environments in which they are expressed. Penetrance is the concept that there are only a proportion of individuals with an expected phenotype expressed based on their common genotype. Although we carry definite physical characteristics and propensities, our physical and emotional environments can determine the likelihood of certain genes to be expressed. Genes differ in what traditionally has been known as expressivity, the extent to which an individual with the gene expresses its trait.

Barbara McClintock won the Noble prize for demonstrating the ability of genes to change within a single life cycle of corn. These "jumping genes," or genetic transpositions, may be important in gene repair and may indicate that the DNA itself is part of a self-regulatory system that relies on other events in the organism for its direction. We know that DNA maintains continuity, but that still does not explain what directs the pattern of organization in the first place.

In neurophysiology, we find the brain is molded by environmental input and the responses of the individual. The result is that the mind and central nervous system are not simply the result of chemical interactions, but are influenced by human interpretation and interactions of will and intent. Their dynamic interaction does not repudiate our basic knowledge of neuronal function; it simply places it once again in the context of our experience of life.

The beauty of the whole story is that most of the great scientists who introduced what we now know as our mechanistic science had vitalistic beliefs. They did not see these principles as contradictory. Johannes Kepler (1571–1630), who described the mathematics for the movement of planets around the sun, was also seeking the position for its origins, that is for the existence of God. Sir Issac Newton (1642–1727), who described gravity and created the science of optics, was a great student of alchemy. In the twentieth century, Friedrich Kekule was revealed the solution to his attempts to find the structure of benzene through a dream of the ouroboros, an archetypal image of a snake biting its own tail and an ancient alchemical symbol of death and renewal. When he applied the concept of a circular or ring structure to benzene, suddenly everything was explained.

Science returns in its complexity to its origins. This is a modern problem. The conflict between empiricism, which viewed the results of treatment more important than the theories of mechanism, and the mechanists who needed an explanation for why the treatment worked for its acceptance, persists today as the major questions for scientific research. Koch's postulate, introduced in 1884, one of the foundations of modern research, states the cause of a disease is capable of being demonstrated by isolating the causal agent in a culture and introducing it into a host. If the new host develops the disease, the causative agent has been proven. This is also the basis for modern therapeutics, demonstrating a cause and the statistical evidence for an effective therapeutic agent to counteract the cause. While critical in the positive developments of allopathic medicine, Koch's postulate has unfortunately also perpetuated a singular methodology of research.

[130]

It is often the nature of healing to have an effect on diseases without any known causal agent. It may come from the act of touch or the technique applied by touch. It may be that medicine is often an excuse for the thirst for attention and caring. Healing is ultimately a larger event than the resolution of the disease itself.

In Revelations, it states that the leaves of the trees are for the healing of nations. But we are separated. We are taught to be separate. We are taught that what we have is ours. It is the disease of independence, of a puritanically influenced society, when we are actually interdependent.

Life remains a unique opportunity. The body works against entropy and self-destruction, developing increasing levels of complexity unfound in inorganic forms. This is the alchemy of our ancestors that is the creative spirit. This is also the alchemy of today, found in the evolving inspiration of human inquiry and knowledge. That innate wisdom is found in everything that breathes.

This is the book of nature. It is the book of life. We depend on something that is larger than our awareness for our sustenance. It is carried through the water and air, the earth and the sun. It is primordial and eternal. It is silent and melodic. That is why we can speak of the spiritual source of disease, without denying the relationship to its physicality. Because our alchemy is the expression of the self, it is expressed through our bodies. Disease can be seen in the revelation of an unfolding mystery as clues in which healing is the solution. We carry it with us as a potentiality at all times.

Vitalism remains in all solutions that acknowledge our limitations and call upon the transpersonal. It may come from our wills or imaginations. It may use the symbolic language of the unconscious. It may come by releasing an old hurt that has held us fixated throughout life. It is the recognition of something we know to be true deep inside. That is why this respect for life and its mysteries is sustained. It is a participatory science in which consciousness and ethics are the focus rather than the outcome. Vitalism arises not out of superstition or holding onto some dogma of an obsolete science but out of a deep sense that what has come before us is still a part of us no matter how sophisticated our knowledge. It is essential so that our ancient selves, our primal and animal nature, our natural wisdom and creativity, are integrated in our minds so that we do not risk the revolt of our own denied selves.

RESOURCES

Abrams, Albert. *Spondylotherapy.* Philopolis Press, San Francisco, 1918.

Amrine, Frederick et al. "Goethe and the Sciences: A Reappraisal." *Boston Studies in the Philosophy of Science,* volume 97. D. Reidel Publishing Company, Dordrecht, 1987.

Bastide, Madeleine. *Signals and Images.* Kluwer Academic Publishers, Dordrecht, 1997.

Bellavite, Paolo and Signorini, Andrea. Homeopathy, *A Frontier in Medical Science.* North Atlantic Books, Berkeley, 1995.

Becker, Robert O. *Cross Currents: the Promise of Electromedicine, the Perils of Electropollution.* Jeremy P. Tarcher, Los Angeles, 1990.

Berman, Morris. *The Reenchantment of the World.* Cornell University Press, Ithaca, 1981.

Bloch, George. *Body and Self: Elements of Human Biology, Behavior, and Health.* William Kaufmann, Los Altos.

Boger, Cyrus M. *Studies in the Philosophy of Healing.* Roy and Company, Bombay, 1964.

Campbell, Joseph. *Spirit and Nature: Papers from the Eranos Yearbooks.* Princeton University Press, Princeton, 1972.

Capra, Fritjof. *The Web of Life.* Anchor Books, New York, 1996.

Clagett, Marshall. *Greek Science in Antiquity.* Abelard-Schuman, New York, 1955.

Clarke, Edwin and Jacyna L.S. *Nineteenth-Century Origins of Neuroscientific Concepts.* University of California, Berkeley, 1987.

Coulter, Harris L. Divided Legacy: *A History of the Schism in Medical Thought.* Wehawken Book Company, Washington DC, 1973.

Cullen, William. *Lectures on Materia Medica.* Thomas Ewing, Dublin, 1773.

Dawson, Adele G. *Health, Happiness and the Pursuit of Herbs.* Stephen Greene Press, Brattleboro, 1980.

Debus, Allen G. *The Chemical Philosophy: Paracelsian Science and Mathematics in the Sixteenth and Seventeenth Centuries.* Science History Publications, New York, 1977.

Delaporte, Francois. *Nature's Second Kingdom: Explorations of Vegetality in the Eighteenth Century.* MIT Press, Cambridge, 1982.

De Telepnef, Basilio. *Paracelsus: A Genius Amidst a Troubled World.* Banton Press, Largs, 1991.

Dobbs, B.J.T. *The Foundations of Newton's Alchemy or, the Hunting of the Greene Lion.* Cambridge University Press, 1975.

Drost-Hansen, W. and Clegg, James S. *Cell-Associated Water.* Academic Press. New York, 1979.

Dubrov, A.P. *The Geomagnetic Field and Life.* Plenum Press, New York, 1978.

Eamon, William. *Science and the Secrets of Nature.* Princeton University Press, Princeton, 1994.

Erickson, Milton H. *The Collected Papers of Milton H. Erickson on Hypnosis.* Irvington Publishers, New York, 1980.

Feher, Michael. *Fragments for a History of the Human Body.* Zone Books, New York, 1989.

Gregory, Richard L. *Mind in Science.* Cambridge University Press, Cambridge, 1981.

Grossinger, Richard. *Planet Medicine: From Stone Age Shamanism to Post-Industrial Healing.* North Atlantic Books, Berkeley, 1980.

Hahnemann, Samuel. *Organon of Medicine 6th edition.* J.P. Tarcher, Los Angeles, 1982.

Hall, Thomas S. *Ideas of Life and Matter.* University of Chicago Press, Chicago, 1969.

Haraway, Donna Jeanne. *Crystals, Fabrics, and Fields: Metaphors of Twentieth-century Developmental Biology.* Yale University Press, New Haven and London, 1976.

Hauschka, Rudolf. *The Nature of Substance.* Vincent Stuart Limited, London, 1966.

Hickman, Mae and Maxine, Guy. *Care of the Wild Feathered and Furred: A Guide to Wildlife Handling and Care.* Unity Press, Santa Cruz, 1973.

Jung, C.G. *Collected Works: Symbols of Transformation.* Princeton University Press, Princeton, 1956.

Kerenyi, C. *Asclepios.* Pantheon Books, New York, 1959.

Issacs, James P. and Lamb, John. *Complementarity in Biology: Organization of Molecular Motion.* John Hopkins Press, Baltimore, 1969.

Kelso, J.A. Scott. *Dynamic Patterns: The Self-organization of Brain and Behavior.* Massachusetts Institute of Technology, Cambridge and London, 1995.

Krishnamurti, Jiddu. *The Awakening of Intelligence.* Harper and Row, New York, 1973.

Kuriyama, Shigehisa. *The Expressiveness of the Body and the Divergence of Greek and Chinese Medicine.* Zone Books, New York, 1999.

Lappe, Marc. *The Tao of Immunology.* Plenum Press, New York, 1997.

Lappe, Marc. *Evolutionary Medicine: Rethinking the Origins of Disease.* Sierra Club Books, San Francisco, 1994.

Lillie, Ralph. *General Biology and the Philosophy of the Organism.* University of Chicago Press, Chicago, 1945.

Lyons, Albert S. and Petrucelli, R. Joseph II. *Medicine An Illustrated History.* Harry N. Abrams, New York, 1978.

MacLeod, G. *The Treatment of Cattle by Homeopathy.* Health Science Press, Essex, 1981. P. Watkins, London, 1919.

Mesmer, F.A. *Mesmerism: A translation of the Original Medical and Scientific Writings of F.A. Mesmer, M.D.* Translated by George J. Bloch, William Kaufmann, Los Angeles, 1980.

Nasr, Sayed Hossein. *Science and Civilization in Islam.* Barnes and Noble, New York, 1968.

Needham, Joseph. *Biochemistry and Morphogenesis.* Cambridge University Press, Cambridge, 1950.

Needham, Joseph. *Science and Civilisation in China.* Cambridge University Press, Cambridge, 1961.

Newman, William R. *Gehennical Fire.* Harvard University Press, Cambridge, 1994.

Pagel, Walter. *Parcelsus: An Introduction to Philosophical Medicine in the Era of the Renaissance.* Karger, Basel, 1982.

Payer, Lynn. *Medicine and Culture.* Henry Holt and Company, New York, 1988.

Pearce, Joseph Chilton. *Evolution's End.* Harper, San Francisco, 1992.

Pelikan, Wilhelm. *The Secrets of Metals.* Anthroposophic Press, Spring Valley, New York, 1973.

Pottenger, Francis Marion. *Symptoms of Visceral Disease.* C.V. Mosby, St. Louis, 1938.

Presman, A.S. *Electromagnetic Fields and Life.* Plenum Press, New York, 1970

Riddle, John M. *Dioscorides on Pharmacy and Medicine.* University of Texas Press, Austin, 1985.

Rilke, Rainier Maria, translated by Norton, Herter. *Letters to a Young Poet.* W.W. Norton, New York, 1934.

Roberts, Herbert A. *The Principles and Art of Cure by Homeopathy.* Health Sciences Press, Rustington, 1942.

Rothenberg, Jerome and Rothenberg, Diane. *Symposium of the Whole: A Range of Discourses Toward and Ethnopoetics.* University of California Press, Berkeley, 1983.

Sarton, George. *A History of Science.* Harvard University Press, Cambridge, 1959.

Sigerist, Henry E., *A History of Medicine.* Oxford University Press, New York, 1961.

Snyder, Gary. *The Real Work: Interviews and Talks 1964 1979.* New Directions Books, New York, 1980.

Solov'ev, V.D. and Bektemirov, T.A., *Interferon: Theory and Applications.* Plenum Press, New York, 1973.

Taussig, Michael. *The Nervous System.* Routledge, New York, 1992.

Tobyn, Graeme. *Culpepper's Medicine: A Practice of Western Holistic Medicine.* Element Books Limited, Shaftesbury, 1997.

Unschuld, Paul U. *Medicine in China: A History of Ideas.* University of California Press, Berkeley, 1985.

Uyldert, Mellie. *Metal Magic.* Turnstone Press Limited, Wellingborough, 1980.

Vogel, Virgil. *American Indian Medicine.* University of Oklahoma Press, Norman, 1970.

Whitaker, Sir Edmund. *A History of the Theories of Aether and Electricity*. Harper Torchbook, New York, 1960.

Whitmont, Edward C. *Psyche and Substance: Essays on Homeopathy in the Light of Jungian Psychology*. North Atlantic Books, Berkeley, 1980.

Winfree, Arthur T. *When Time Breaks Down: The Three-Dimensional Dynamics of Electrochemical Waves and Cardiac Arythmias*. Princeton University Press, Princeton, 1987.

Wood, Matthew. *The Magical Staff: The Vitalist Tradition in Western Medicine*. North Atlantic Books, Berkeley, 1992.

Wright-Hubbard, Elizabeth. *Homeopathy as Art and Science*. Beaconsfield Publishers, Beaconsfield, 1990.

Yabrov, Alexander A. *Interferon and Nonspecific Resistance*. Human Sciences Press, New York, 1980.

Zaren, Ananda. *Core Elements of the Materia Medica of the Mind Volume I*. Ulrich Burgdorf Homoeopathic Publishing House, Germany, 1994.